MW01716465

Instructor's Guide for

Concept Mapping: A Critical-Thinking Approach to Care Planning

Instructor's Guide for

Concept Mapping: A Critical-Thinking Approach to Care Planning

Pamela McHugh Schuster, RN, PhD
Professor of Nursing

Youngstown State University
Youngstown, Ohio

F.A. Davis Company • Philadelphia

F. A. Davis Company
1915 Arch Street
Philadelphia, PA 1910
www.fadavis.com

ISBN: 0-8036-0981-7

Printed in the United States of America

Last digit indicates print number: 10 9 8 7 6

As new scientific information becomes available through basic and clinical research, recommended treatments and drug therapies undergo changes. The author(s) and publisher have done everything possible to make this book accurate, up to date, and in accord with accepted standards at the time of publication. The author(s), editors, and publisher are not responsible for errors or omissions or for consequences from application of the book, and make no warranty, expressed or implied, in regard to the contents of the book. Any practice described in this book should be applied by the reader in accordance with professional standards of care used in regard to the unique circumstances that may apply in each situation. The reader is advised always to check product information (package inserts) for changes and new information regarding dose and contraindications before administering any drug. Caution is especially urged when using new or infrequently ordered drugs.

Contents

Chapter 1

‘Twas the Night before Clinical . . .

Overview

For nearly 15 years, I taught care planning using the same multicolumn format that virtually all other nursing instructors used. You know the one. It has columns for nursing diagnoses, goals, outcome objectives, interventions with rationales, and evaluations. But I was frustrated. I wanted my students to gather information on assigned patients ahead of time and come to the unit prepared to care for them. Using the standard care plan format, however, was a less-than-satisfying process.

First of all, as you know, students cannot be realistically expected to write up every actual and potential nursing diagnosis for each of their patients. In addition, although faculty members universally prefer that students plan their nursing care ahead of time, the fact is that much of the work on column-based care plans can be done only after the clinical day is over. Even then, students typically have a difficult time summarizing patient data, connecting patient problems logically, and gathering information into a succinct and comprehensive plan. Plus, it takes a long time to write up each objective, intervention, and rationale.

On a day when I was particularly frustrated by my students’ inability to use their care plans to reason their way through the priorities of a patient’s care, I told them to get a blank sheet of paper and write the reason for the patient’s admission in the center of the page. Then I encouraged them to arrange all of the patient’s other problems in a spoke-like fashion around the main reason for their health-care admission. I told them to group the assessment data, treatments, and medications under the problems. What a difference! The students used critical thinking to organize the data they had collected about the patient’s problems, and they then began to better understand the relationships among those data. From there, they developed wonderful ideas regarding patient-care planning and implementation of effective care. Their performance in the clinical setting quickly improved, and they were very pleased with themselves and the care they provided. So was I.

I was so pleased at the progress my students were making that I described what I was doing to a colleague with a psychiatric nursing background. She told me that my students were doing concept mapping. Reviewing the literature confirmed that the theoretical basis for concept mapping originated from assimilation theory and meaningful learning theory credited to J. Novak and D. Gowin (*Learning How to Learn,* Cambridge University Press, 1984) and to D. Ausubel (*Educational Psychology: A Cognitive View,* Holt, Rinehart, & Winston, 1978). Although I had discovered nothing new, the development and application of concept mapping for nursing students was clearly an exciting and innovative prospect.

Since I first discovered the application to nursing care planning and began writing and speaking about concept map care plans at conferences and workshops, concept map care plans have been adopted by many faculty and used in numerous health-care settings to organize and individualize comprehensive nursing care, increase learning, and improve clinical performance. Students come to clinical sessions with a comprehensive care plan in hand. Faculty can quickly evaluate concept map care plans to see if students have identified major patient problems, correlated significant data, and identified appropriate nursing interventions just by glancing at the diagram and intervention lists.

In addition, there is much less paperwork for students and decreased time faculty must spend reading and grading clinical care plans. Faculty usually spend many hours grading column-based nursing care plans each week. And the worst part is that students typically copy column-based care plan information straight from a standardized care planning book. How much critical thinking can that require?

I have found that both students and faculty who use the concept map method of care planning are very pleased with the results. Concept maps are specific to the patient, are concise, and are organized. They save time and energy, and they decrease the tedious paperwork needed for column-based care plans. Concept maps allow a holistic view of the patient, and they cover all patient problems, which means that students can better learn to integrate and understand the relationships among patient problems. Standardized nursing care plans can be found on many nursing units and in many textbooks. As nursing educators, our focus should be on customizing care plans, using time more efficiently, and increasing learning by helping students better organize and plan.

Most of students' work on a concept map care plan is completed before clinical, with little work left to be done except completing the evaluation components of the care plan and evaluating their own performance. In developing concept map care plans, students do not have to spend many hours developing a column-based care plan after completing the clinical experience. Instead, their time has been spent preparing ahead of time for patient care. Students have reported the time spent has been worthwhile, because they can see their own clinical progress and use information in the care plan to actually give patient care. Nursing care plans can realistically be done before the clinical day, and then used during the clinical day.

Reviewing Chapter 1

This chapter gives the student an overview of the components of concept map care planning. It also addresses the relationship between care planning and standards of care. Students commonly have trouble understanding the relationship between nursing process, care planning, and standards of care. It can be difficult for them to remember that everything in health care is based on standards of care established by health-care providers, government agencies, and insurance companies. The standards aimed at cutting costs while maintaining quality have led to a state of turmoil in health care. Students in nursing programs must have this understanding very early in their education because the financial aspects of care impact directly on the type of care planning that students will be doing. It is also important to introduce the concept of managed care as one means to control costs and maintain quality of patient care.

Teaching Tips

1. Start with an overview of the basic steps in developing a concept map care plan.
2. Develop a skeleton diagram of health problems. Place the reason the person requires health care in the center of the diagram, with all other identified problems radiating from it like spokes on a wheel.
3. Analyze and categorize specific assessment data under problems.
4. Indicate relationships among problems.
5. Develop patient-specific goals, outcomes, and interventions.
6. Evaluate actual patient responses to nursing interventions and summarize clinical impressions.

I've found that students who are first learning the concept map care planning process may benefit from having boxes drawn for them to fill in. The blank boxes provide a structural outline for the concept map care plan process. A word processing program can be used to draw boxes and lines.

Step 1

In the first Step, students determine the patient's key problems (also known as the concepts) based on the data collected. After placing the patient's reason for seeking health care (often a medical diagnosis) in the center of the page, they should arrange the patient's major problems (based on assessment data) around the center problem like the spokes of a wheel. A blank version of this arrangement appears on the next page.

Step 2

In the second Step, have students add clinical data to the appropriate problem boxes, including abnormal physical assessment findings, treatments, medications, IV therapy, abnormal diagnostic and lab tests, medical history, and the patient's emotional and pain state. Also, have them identify key assessments related to the patient's reason for health care (chief medical diagnosis/surgical procedure). These key assessment items are written in the center box. If a student doesn't know where to place certain data, suggest he puts it in a separate box off to the side of the main map. The map on page 7 shows such a box.

Step 3

In Step 3, have the students draw lines between related problems and number the problems to prioritize them. Finally have students label each problem with a nursing diagnosis.

Step 4

In this step, students identify goals, outcomes, and interventions on a form such as the one shown on page 8.

Step 5

During clinical sessions, student evaluate patient responses.

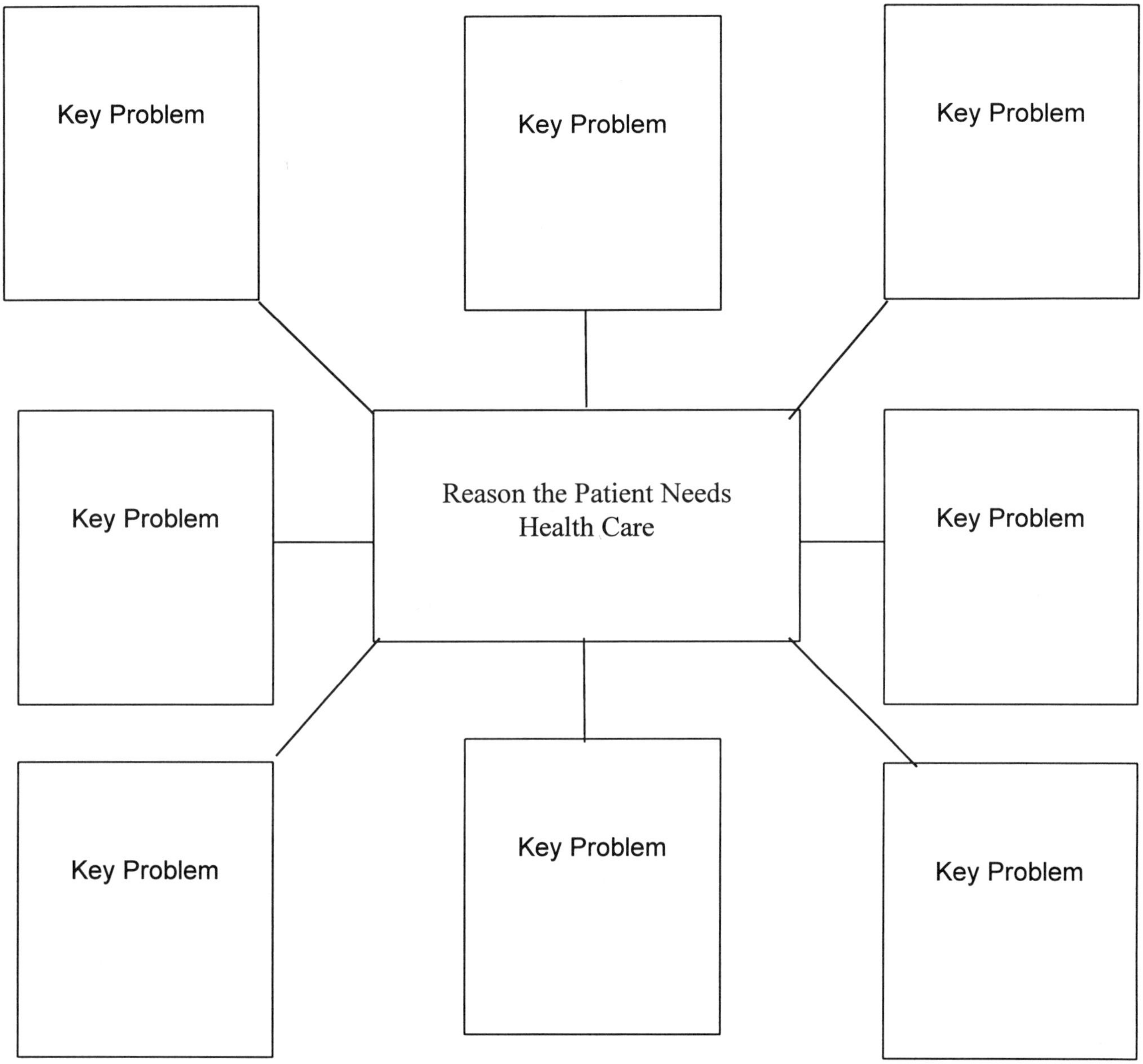
Key Problem
Key Problem
Key Problem
Key Problem
Reason the Patient Needs Health Care
Key Problem
Key Problem
Key Problem
Key Problem

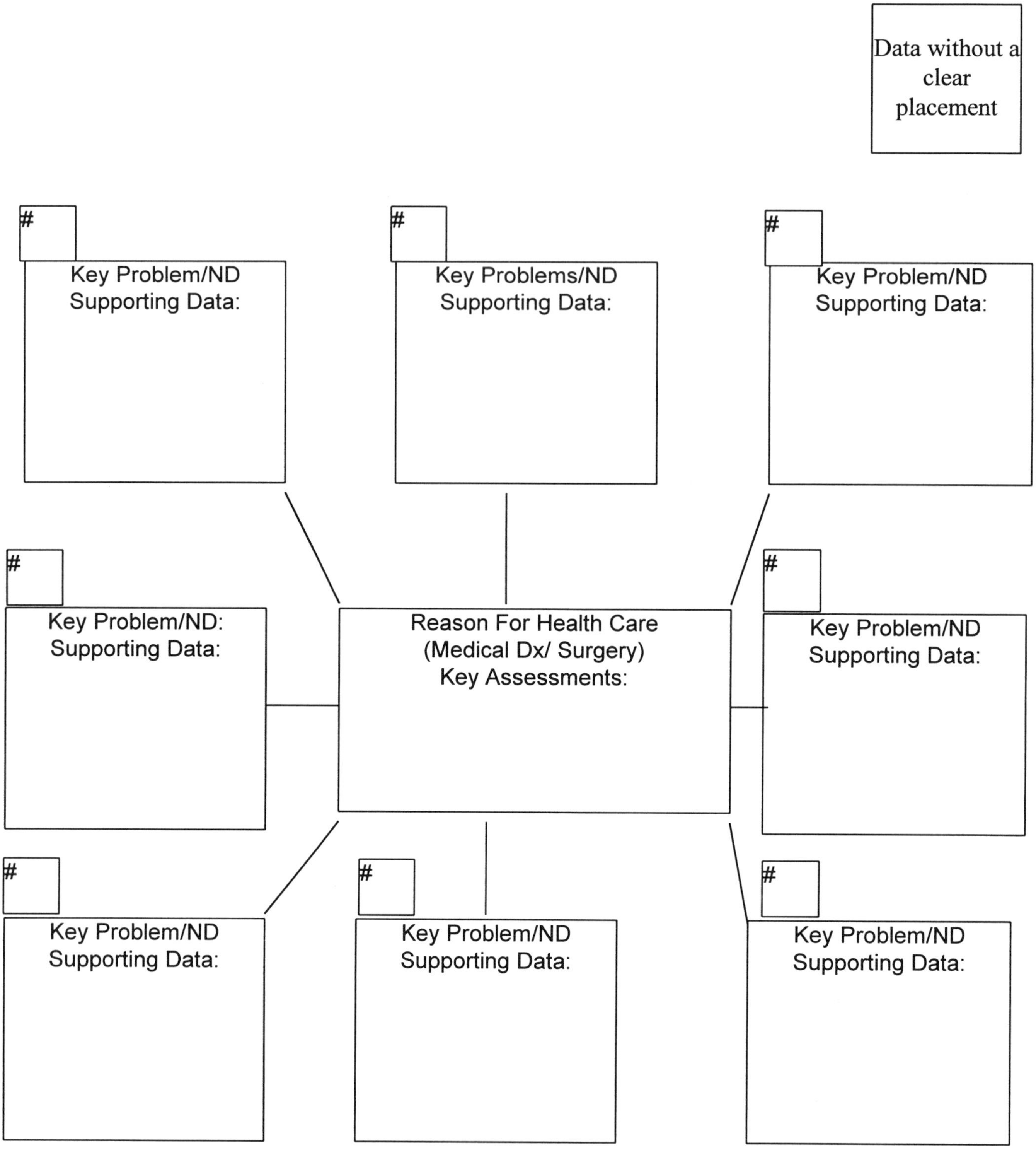
Data without a clear placement
#
Key Problem/ND
Supporting Data:
#
Key Problems/ND
Supporting Data:
#
Key Problem/ND
Supporting Data:
#
Key Problem/ND:
Supporting Data:
Reason For Health Care
(Medical Dx/ Surgery)
Key Assessments:
#
Key Problem/ND
Supporting Data:
#
Key Problem/ND
Supporting Data:
#
Key Problem/ND
Supporting Data:
#
Key Problem/ND
Supporting Data:

Problem No. 1:
General goal:

Behavioral Outcome Objective(s): The patient will. . .

on the day of care.

Nursing interventions	Patient responses (evaluation)
1.	1.
2.	2.
3.	3.
4.	4.
5.	5.
6.	6.
7.	7.
8.	8.

Summarize impressions of patient progress toward outcomes:

Problem No. 2:
General goal:

Behavioral Outcome Objective(s): The patient will. . .

on the day of care.

Nursing interventions	Patient responses
1.	1.
2.	2.
3.	3.
4.	4.
5.	5.
6.	6.
7.	7.
8.	8.

Summarize Impressions of patient progress toward outcomes:

One point is important to emphasize as you give students a general overview of concept map care planning: Make the connection between the diagram used in Steps 1, 2, and 3 with the American Nurses Association Social Policy Statement that says, "The focus of nursing practice is on human responses to health states." The concept map represents the health state, centrally located, as the reason for seeking health care, and the human responses to the health state, which are the key problems surrounding the reason for seeking health care.

Rationales for Learning Activities

Chapter 1 gives students a basic understanding of concept map care planning and teaches how to do a concept map care plan. The learning activities for this chapter are designed for students to use standards of care during clinical practice. Students commonly have difficulty understanding the relationship between nursing process, care planning, and standards of care. They need to locate and use sample standardized care plans, clinical pathways, and clinical procedures along with the individualized concept map care plan to give patient care. The purpose of a post-conference session with a case manager, discharge planner, or utilization review person is for the student to recognize the emphasis on controlling costs in health-care settings while at the same time providing quality care, in accordance with standards of care.

Chapter 2

Gathering Clinical Data: The Framework for Concept map Care Plans

Chapter 2 is focused on the first standard of practice of the American Nurses Association—gathering and recording real clinical data. It is important to guide students in the collection of clinical evidence pertaining to a patient's health status. Make it clear that collecting accurate clinical data is the most important thing nurses do. This is because a clear understanding of a patient's problems and the ability to make sound clinical judgments both emanate from accurate and complete data collection.

Although nurses do not have the knowledge and skill to develop treatment plans for all problems, if they recognize the existence of a problem based on the evidence collected, they can then refer the patient to another health-care provider for care of the problem, as needed. This is important to emphasize when teaching. Gradually, nursing students do develop the knowledge and skills to develop and implement plans to solve many problems. But there will always be problems that other health-care providers must solve. Learning who is responsible and accountable to whom and learning to refer problems to appropriate members of the health-care team are crucial for students to learn early in the nursing program.

Teaching Tips

Although patients' reasons for seeking health care vary widely, students must learn to collect certain basic data from them regardless of the health-care setting where they are being treated. Begin with an overview of the basic characteristics of data that must be gathered in any clinical setting. Specifically, the student must gather data about the following:

- Patient's reason for seeking care and current health problems
- Health history
- Physical assessment data
- Treatments
- Medications
- Intravenous (IV) therapy
- Diet
- Activity level
- Diagnostic tests
- Laboratory values
- Growth and development
- Emotional state

A specific database to guide the collection of data is needed in each clinical setting. The database used as an example in this book is designed for patients in acute-care settings and students in foundations and medical-surgical courses. It is a basic guide. Each component of the form is specifically numbered so that students can refer to written descriptions of what information is collected, where it is usually found in the documented patient records, and why it is important to collect that particular type of data. I have always gone over this information verbally with students in lecture and then again on the clinical units; I still recommend doing so. However, these written explanations can be quite helpful as a teaching-learning tool and as a reference to data collection. A blank patient database form is included at the end of this chapter.

Introduce students gradually to data collection so they will not be overwhelmed. For example, if students have not yet learned principles of fluid and electrolyte balance and IV therapy, they may only be required to note the patient has an IV but not to collect the specific details of solution type, rate of administration, or assessment of the site. Likewise, they may not be expected to collect information about laboratory tests until they have studied these topics during the course. Students who have not had pharmacology and medication administration should not be expected to assess data regarding medications. Students who have not yet learned neurological assessments should not be expected to collect all data associated with neurological status. However, all students in patient-care settings would be expected to note the patient's level of alertness and to assess confusion, because these can impact basic safety.

In foundations, students typically begin by learning about safety and skin care, and they learn falls risk assessment and skin assessment. Interventions include safety in handling patients, preventing falls, and using good body mechanics and hygiene. In foundations courses, I have students complete the hospital's standardized falls and skin assessments for their patients in addition to the basic database. It is important for students to learn to use standardized assessment forms in conjunction with the clinical database for collection of data. Samples of a standardized falls and skin assessment are included in this chapter. If students in a clinical course have not yet learned many aspects of patient assessment and data collection, they will first learn basic concepts of hygiene, immobility, and safety principles and their applications to care planning. These students should be focused on the use of standardized assessments for falls and hygiene and should formulate a basic care map of hygiene, immobility, and safety needs for the patient.

Even though students have not yet studied all aspects of the assessment that appear on the basic patient profile database, it is important to review the entire data collection form early in the term so that students are aware of what they need to accomplish by term's end. Such a review guides students to pay attention when something is happening on a clinical unit, even though they have not yet learned about it. For example, if a nurse will be in the room monitoring IV therapy for a patient assigned to one of your students, the student should know to observe how the nurse monitors the patient's IV therapy. I have often been asked to describe how to "level" concept maps throughout a curriculum. Each course focuses on assessment of progressively more intricate data within a variety of health-care settings.

The patient database is the key to developing an accurate diagram of patient problems. Be sure to emphasize that concept maps are developed based on real clinical data. Focus students on actual, not potential, clinical problems based on clinical evidence that can be realistically collected the night before or the morning of the clinical experience. It is important to note that this database contains only the information that could be obtained either the night before clinical or the beginning of the shift. There are very few psycho-social-cultural assessment data in this initial assessment. This is purposely done so that students are not overwhelmed and can focus on specific aspects of data collection to formulate the initial concept map. Psycho-social-cultural assessment data is very important, but students need time to interact with patients to collect this form of data. Collection of psycho-social-cultural data is described in Chapter 6, and a tool for collecting these data is provided in that chapter as well.

Rationales for Learning Activities

It is the intent of these activities to carefully guide and support students through the collection of data until they feel comfortable completing the collection on their own. When clinical faculty orient students to clinical units, they typically show students where all the data can be found to complete the basic database and where to obtain their assignments. It helps if students have clinical faculty available to guide the initial gathering of patient data, because although they have been oriented to units, they are commonly nervous, forget where to find everything, and are frustrated by all the abbreviations and unclear, handwritten documentation about patients. I always make it a point to be available on the units as students begin to collect data for the first time at each new clinical site.

An important part of data collection is receiving patient status reports from staff and learning to be assertive and ask questions. Students are commonly not assertive and are uncomfortable interrupting busy staff nurses. Students need specific directions regarding the nature of accountability and responsibility of all staff with whom they come in contact, but especially the staff nurses who are their cover nurses. They need to know how and when to approach staff with questions about patient care. This is further discussed in Chapter 5, which is focused on implementation and evaluation of nursing care.

In addition, students need specific instructions for introducing themselves to patients the day before clinical. Many students are bashful about introducing themselves to patients and families. It is important to have students do this activity so they recognize that they can do a brief cognitive/emotional assessment in just 5 minutes of interacting with a patient.

PATIENT PROFILE DATABASE

ADMISSION INFORMATION

Student Name ....

1 Date of Care:	2 Patient Initials:	3 Age: (face sheet)	3 Growth and Development:	4 Sex: (face sheet)	5 Admission Date: (face sheet)

6 **Reason for Hospitalization** (face sheet):

7 **Medical Diagnoses:** (present diagnoses, past diagnoses; physician's History and Physical notes in chart; nursing intake assessment and Kardex)

8 **Surgical Procedures** (consent forms and Kardex):

9 ADVANCE DIRECTIVES (NURSE'S ADMISSION ASSESSMENTS):

Living will: ☐ yes ☐ no | Power of attorney: ☐ yes ☐ no | Do not resuscitate (DNR) order (Kardex): ☐ yes ☐ no

10 LABORATORY DATA

Test	Norms	On admission	Current value	Test	Norms	On admission	Current value
White blood cells				Potassium			
Differential				Blood Glucose			
Hemoglobin				Glycohemoglobin			
Hematocrit				Cholesterol			
Platelets				Low-density lipoproteins			
Prothrombin time				Urine analysis			
International normalized ratio							
Activated partial thromboplastin time				Other abnormal			

11 DIAGNOSTIC TESTS

Chest x-ray:	EKG:	Other abnormal reports:
Other:	Other:	Other:

12 MEDICATIONS

List medications and times of administration (medication administration record and check the drawer in the carts for spelling):

Medication/Time of Administration	Medication/Time of Administration	Medication/Time of Administration

ALLERGIES / PAIN

13 Allergies (medication administration records):	14 When was the last pain medication given? (medication administration record):
14 Where is the pain? (nurse's notes):	14 How much pain is the patient in on a scale from 0 – 10? (nurse's notes, flow sheet):

TREATMENTS

15 Treatments (Kardex):	16 Support services (Kardex):	17 Consultations (Kardex):

18 DIET / FLUIDS

Type of Diet (Kardex):	Restrictions (Kardex):	Gag reflex intact: ☐ yes ☐ no	Appetite: Breakfast ____ %	Lunch ____ %	Supper ____ %

Circle Those Problems That Apply:

Fluid intake: 24 hours (flow sheet)	• Problems: swallowing, chewing, dentures (nurse's notes) • Needs assistance with feeding (nurse's notes) • Nausea or vomiting (nurse's notes)
Tube feedings: type and rate (Kardex)	• Overhydrated or dehydrated (evaluate total intake and output on flow sheet) • Belching • Other: ____________

19 INTRAVENOUS FLUIDS (IV therapy record)

Type and rate:	IV dressing dry, no edema, redness of site: ☐ yes ☐ no	Other:

20 ELIMINATION (flow sheet)

Last bowel movement:	24-hour urine output:	Foley/condom catheter: ☐ yes ☐ no

Circle Those Problems That Apply:

• Bowel:	constipation	diarrhea	flatus	incontinence	belching
• Urinary:	hesitancy	frequency	burning	incontinence	odor
• Other: ____________					

21 ACTIVITY (Kardex, flow sheet)

Ability to walk (gait):	Type of activity orders:	Use of assistive devices: cane, walker, crutches, prosthesis:	Falls-risk assessment rating:
No. of side rails required (flow sheet):	Restraints (flow sheet): ☐ yes ☐ no	Weakness: ☐ yes ☐ no	Trouble sleeping (nurse's notes): ☐ yes ☐ no

PHYSICAL ASSESSMENT DATA

22 BP (flow sheet):	22 TPR (flow sheet):	23 Height: ______ Weight: ______ (nursing intake assessments)

REVIEW OF SYSTEMS

Write WNL (within normal limits) if normal and describe abnormalities in space provided: (check nurses' notes and shift assessments for the latest information you can get)

PATIENT PROFILE DATABASE *(cont.)*

24 NEUROLOGICAL/MENTAL STATUS: ______

LOC: alert and oriented to person, place, time (A&O x 3) confused, etc.	Speech: clear, appropriate/inappropriate

Motor: ROM x 4 extremities	Sensation: 4 extremities	Pupils: PERRLA	Sensory deficits for vision/hearing/taste/smell

25 MUSCULOSKELETAL SYSTEM: ______

Bones, joints, muscles (fractures, contractures, arthritis, spinal curvatures, etc.):	Extremity circulation checks (pulses, temperature, sensation, edema):
Ted hose/plexi pulses/compression devices: type:	Casts, splint, collar, brace:

26 CARDIOVASCULAR SYSTEM: ______

Pulses (radial, pedal) (to touch or with Doppler):	Capillary refill (<3 s): ☐ yes ☐ no	Edema, pitting vs. nonpitting:
Neck vein (distention):	Sounds: S_1, S_2, regular, irregular:	Any chest pain:

27 RESPIRATORY SYSTEM: ______

Depth, rate, rhythm:	Use of accessory muscles:	Cyanosis:	Sputum: color, amount:	Cough: productive, nonproductive:	Breath sounds: clear, rales, wheezes:

Use of oxygen: nasal cannula, mask, trach collar:	Flow rate of oxygen:	Oxygen humidification: ☐ yes ☐ no	Pulse oximeter: ______% oxygen saturation	Smoking: ☐ yes ☐ no

28 GASTROINTESTINAL SYSTEM: ______

Abdominal pain, tenderness, guarding; distention, soft, firm:	Bowel sounds x 4 quadrants:	NG tube: describe drainage:

Ostomy: describe stoma site and stools:	Other:

29 SKIN AND WOUNDS: ______

Color, turgor:	Rash, bruises:	Describe wounds (size, location):	Edges approximated: ☐ yes ☐ no	Type of wound drains:
Characteristics of drainage:	Dressings (clean, dry, intact):	Sutures, staples, steri-strips, other:	Risk for decubitus ulcer assessment rating:	Other:

30 EYES, EARS, NOSE, THROAT (EENT): ______

Eyes: redness, drainage, edema. ptosis	Ears: drainage	Nose: redness, drainage, edema	Throat: sore

PSYCHOSOCIAL AND CULTURAL ASSESSMENT:

31 Religious preference (face sheet):	32 Marital status (face sheet):	33 Health-care benefits and insurance (face sheet):	34 Occupation (face sheet):	35 Emotional state (nurse's notes):

Additional information to obtain from clinical units the night before clinical specific to your patient's diagnosis:

Standardized falls-risk assessment: ☐ yes ☐ no	Pressure ulcer assessment: ☐ yes ☐ no	Standardized skin assessment: ☐ yes ☐ no	Standardized nursing care plans: ☐ yes ☐ no	Clinical pathways: ☐ yes ☐ no	Patient education materials: ☐ yes ☐ no

BRADEN SCALE >>> FOR PREDICTING PRESSURE SORE RISK

Patient's Name:	Evaluator's Name:	Date of Assessment:

	1	2	3	4
SENSORY PERCEPTION Ability to respond meaningfully to pressure-related discomfort	**Completely limited:** Unresponsive (does not moan, flinch, or grasp) to painful stimuli, due to diminished level of consciousness or sedation, OR limited ability to feel pain over most of the body surface.	**Very Limited:** Responds only to painful stimuli. Cannot communicate discomfort except by moaning or restlessness, OR has a sensory impairment which limits the ability to feel pain or discomfort over 1/2 of the body.	**Slightly Limited:** Responds to verbal commands but cannot always communicate discomfort or need to be turned, OR has a sensory impairment which limits ability to feel pain or discomfort in 1 or 2 extremities.	**No Impairment:** Responds to verbal commands. Has no sensory deficit which would limit ability to feel or voice pain or discomfort.
MOISTURE Degree to which skin is exposed to moisture	**Constantly Moist:** Skin is kept moist almost constantly by perspiration, urine, etc. Dampness is detected every time patient is moved or turned.	**Moist:** Skin is often but not always moist. Linen must be changed at least once a shift.	**Occasionally Moist:** Skin is occasionally moist, requiring an extra linen change approximately once a day.	**No Impairment:** Responds to verbal commands. Has no sensory deficit which would limit ability to feel or voice pain or discomfort.
ACTIVITY Degree of physical activity	**Bedfast:** Confined to bed.	**Chairfast:** Ability to walk severely limited or nonexistent. Cannot bear own weight and/or must be assisted into chair or wheelchair.	**Walks Occasionally:** Walks occasionally during day but for very short distances, with or without assistance. Spends majority of each shift in bed or chair.	**Walks Frequently:** Walks outside the room at least twice a day and inside room at least once every 2 hours during walking hours.
MOBILITY Ability to change and control body position	**Completely Immobile:** Does not make even slight changes in body or extremity position without assistance.	**Very Limited:** Makes occasional slight changes in body or extremity position but unable to make frequent or significant changes independently.	**Slightly Limited:** Makes frequent though slight changes in body or extremity position independently.	**No Limitations:** Makes major and frequent changes in position without assistance.
NUTRITION Usual food intake pattern	**Very Poor:** Never eats a complete meal. Rarely eats more than 1/3 of any food offered. Eats 2 servings or less of protein (meat or dairy products) per day. Takes fluids poorly. Does not take a liquid dietary supplement, OR is NPO and/or maintained on clear liquids or IVs for more than 5 days.	**Probably Inadequate:** Rarely eats a complete meal and generally eats only about 1/2 of any food offered. Protein intake includes 3 servings of meat or dairy products per day. Occasionally will take a dietary supplement, OR receives less than optimum amount of liquid diet or tube feeding.	**Adequate:** Eats over half of meals. Eats a total of 4 servings of protein (meat, dairy products) each day. Occasionally will refuse a meal, but will usually take a supplement if offered, OR is on a tube feeding or TPN regimen, which probably meets most of nutritional needs.	**Excellent:** Eats most of every meal. Never refuses a meal. Usually eats a total of 4 or more servings of meat and dairy products. Occasionally eats between meals. Does not require supplementation.
FRICTION AND SHEAR	**Problem:** Requires moderate to maximum assistance in moving. Complete lifting without sliding against sheets is impossible. Frequently slides down in bed or chair, requiring frequent repositioning with maximum assistance. Spasticity, contractures, or agitation leads to almost constant friction.	**Potential Problem:** Moves feebly or requires minimum assistance. During a move skin probably slides to some extent against the sheets, chair, restraints, or other devices. Maintains relatively good position in chair or bed most of the time but occasionally slides down.	**No Apparent Problem:** Moves in bed and in chair independently and has sufficient muscle strength to lift up completely during move. Maintains good position in bed or chair at all times.	

RISK FOR FALLS ASSESSMENT

DIRECTIONS: Place an "x" in front of elements that apply to your patient. Based on the assessment, check whatever applies to the patient. A patient for whom you place four or more "x" marks is at risk for falling

GENERAL DATA

___ Age over 60
___ History of falls before admission
___ Postoperative/admitted for operation
___ Smoker

PHYSICAL CONDITION

___ Dizziness/imbalance
___ Unsteady gait
___ Diseases/other problems effecting weight-bearing joints
___ Weakness
___ Paresis
___ Seizure disorder
___ Impairment of vision
___ Impairment of hearing
___ Diarrhea
___ Urinary frequency

MEDICATIONS

___ Diuretics or diuretic effects
___ Hypotensive or CNS suppressants drugs
___ Postoperative/admitted for operation (e.g., narcotic, sedative, psychotropic, hypnotic, tranquilizer, antihypertensive, antidepressant)
___ Medication that increases GI motility

AMBULATORY DEVICES USED

___ Cane
___ Crutches
___ Walker
___ Wheelchair
___ Geriatric (geri) chair
___ Braces

MENTAL STATUS

___ Confusion/disorientation
___ Impaired memory or judgment
___ Inability to understand or follow directions

Chapter 3

Concept Mapping: Grouping Clinical Data in a Meaningful Manner

Once students have practiced collecting data and understand why they need to collect the data identified in the patient profile database, they are ready to develop the concept map diagrams. Students use critical thinking and apply knowledge to accurately group data under the correct general problems. They use the concept map format to literally *organize* their thoughts about the patient. As a result, you can "see" into the minds of students and easily recognize those who understand a patient's care needs from those who are having difficulty.

Teaching Tips

It is very important to teach students in foundations courses a sequence for effectively researching information about the patient data. I recommend the following sequence to my students.

1. Medications and IV fluids

Instruct students to look up drugs and IV fluids first and then list them under problems they have identified. Medication administration is one of the most dangerous tasks for nurses—so I ask students to list these first when their minds are freshest as they prepare the map.

2. Laboratory and diagnostic tests

Instruct students to identify the relationships between any tests and medications that are being administered. Students must realize there is a direct relationship between tests and medications being ordered. Chapter 2 will be a helpful reference to students for many of the common tests.

3. Diet

Instruct the student to relate the patient's diet to her reason for seeking health care. Chapter 2 will be helpful as a reference for many typical diets.

4. Medical diagnoses

Last, but certainly not least, is looking up information for the medical diagnoses and surgical procedures. Students may get overwhelmed by this step because they need to review disease symptoms, etiology, complications, typical treatments, prognosis, and nursing implications of the disease.

The level of knowledge expected of a student in foundations will depend on whether the student has yet had a course in pathophysiology. A reference such as *Taber's Cyclopedic Medical Dictionary* (F.A. Davis) includes all the information needed on many common diagnoses so that even foundations students who have not yet had pathophysiology can begin to consider all aspects of care related to the disease.

In addition, students should review standardized care plans and critical pathways they have located at the clinical facilities. They can also review care plans provided in a care plan book. It is also helpful for students to use a basic medical-surgical textbook as a reference, even in foundations courses.

5. Skin and falls assessments

Have students complete the skin and falls assessments using standardized forms from the facility they will be using for their clinical experience, or have them complete the standardized forms provided in this book.

Building the Concept Map

After giving students some pointers on how to effectively look up information on medications, IVs, tests, diet, medical diagnoses, and surgical procedures, focus your teaching on Steps 1, 2, and 3 of building the concept map. Review each step before having students practice developing diagrams.

Step 1. Develop the skeleton diagram.

Have students write down the patient's key problems based on the data they collected and wrote on the patient profile database. Tell them to center the reason the patient sought health care (commonly a medical diagnosis or surgical procedure) on a blank page. Next, tell them to list the major problems they have identified based on the assessment data collected. This activity can be done on the board or using the blank forms provided in this instructor's manual. The problems should radiate out from the center problem like spokes on a wheel.

Step 2. Analyze and categorize specific patient assessment data and identify key ongoing assessments.

Next, ask students to support the identified problems with abnormal clinical data obtained from their assessments and written down on the patient profile database. They should write each piece of abnormal data under a problem they have identified. This includes abnormal physical assessment findings, treatments, medications, IV fluids, abnormal diagnostic and lab tests, medical history, and the patient's emotional state and pain.

Tell students to write only facts based on clinical evidence. They should not write any potential problems. They should not write the normal data. Of course, this does not mean that students should not consider potential problems and normal data. However, writing normal data and potential problems will take up too much room on the map, and it will confuse the process of focusing on critical thinking about actual patient problems and categorizing evidence to support those problems.

The next phase of Step 2 is to identify and list key assessments that are related to the reason for seeking health care. Tell students to put the key assessments in the center box of the map under the reason for health care. One look at the key assessments and you will be able to tell if the student has identified the most critical ongoing assessments pertinent to the reason for seeking health care. You will easily see what students think are the most important aspects of assessment based on the information they have obtained about a specific patient. This aspect of the concept map care plan is extremely beneficial in the clinical preconference setting where you will be able to easily identify what the student believes should be the primary assessment concerns throughout the clinical day.

Step 3: Identify relationships between problems and labeling nursing diagnoses.

Now have the students draw lines between related problems. It helps if they use a contrasting color of ink as they make the connections. Critical thinking is needed to identify relationships among problems, and you will be able to clearly see by viewing the diagram whether a student has the cognitive knowledge to make appropriate relationships among problems. Students should be able to verbally state the reasons why they indicated relationships among problems. If they have not identified relationships or they cannot give rationales, I have them write them out for subsequent assignments.

Next in Step 2, have the students number problems on the diagram and prioritize them. Typically, the problems with the most data under them or the most lines drawn to them will be the priority problems.

Last, have students label the problems with a nursing diagnostic label approved by the North American Nursing Diagnosis Association (NANDA). Appendixes A, B, and C of the main text will help students to complete this task. The diagnoses are arranged by Maslow's Hierarchy (Appendix A) and Gordon's Functional Patterns (Appendix B), two common frameworks for categorizing types of diagnoses. Appendix C contains NANDA diagnostic labels alphabetized by noun, with definitions for certain labels that are not self-explanatory.

This labeling step is purposely left until the end of the process because many students tend to want to label a problem without first considering all of the factual data. The student's diagnostic accuracy is much improved by labeling last. Many faculty prefer to teach about nursing diagnoses using the three-part nursing diagnosis approach:

1. Name the diagnosis.
2. Establish the "related to" statement (etiology, or what has caused the problem).

3. Add “as evidenced by” (clinical manifestations)..

This process has been beneficial in helping students to critically analyze data, and it could be integrated into the classroom discussion of making accurate nursing diagnoses.

Rationales for Learning Activities

Students need to practice developing concept map diagrams using real patient data so they can have experience in analyzing and categorizing data before going out on their own. Completed Steps 1, 2, and 3 of concept map diagrams of the scenario of a surgical patient with a mastectomy and a surgical patient with a knee replacement have been included in this instructor’s guide. One of the scenarios could be completed with the entire group on a blackboard, whereas the other could be given as a homework assignment. Note that concept maps may vary in appearance, but students are expected to include all abnormal data.

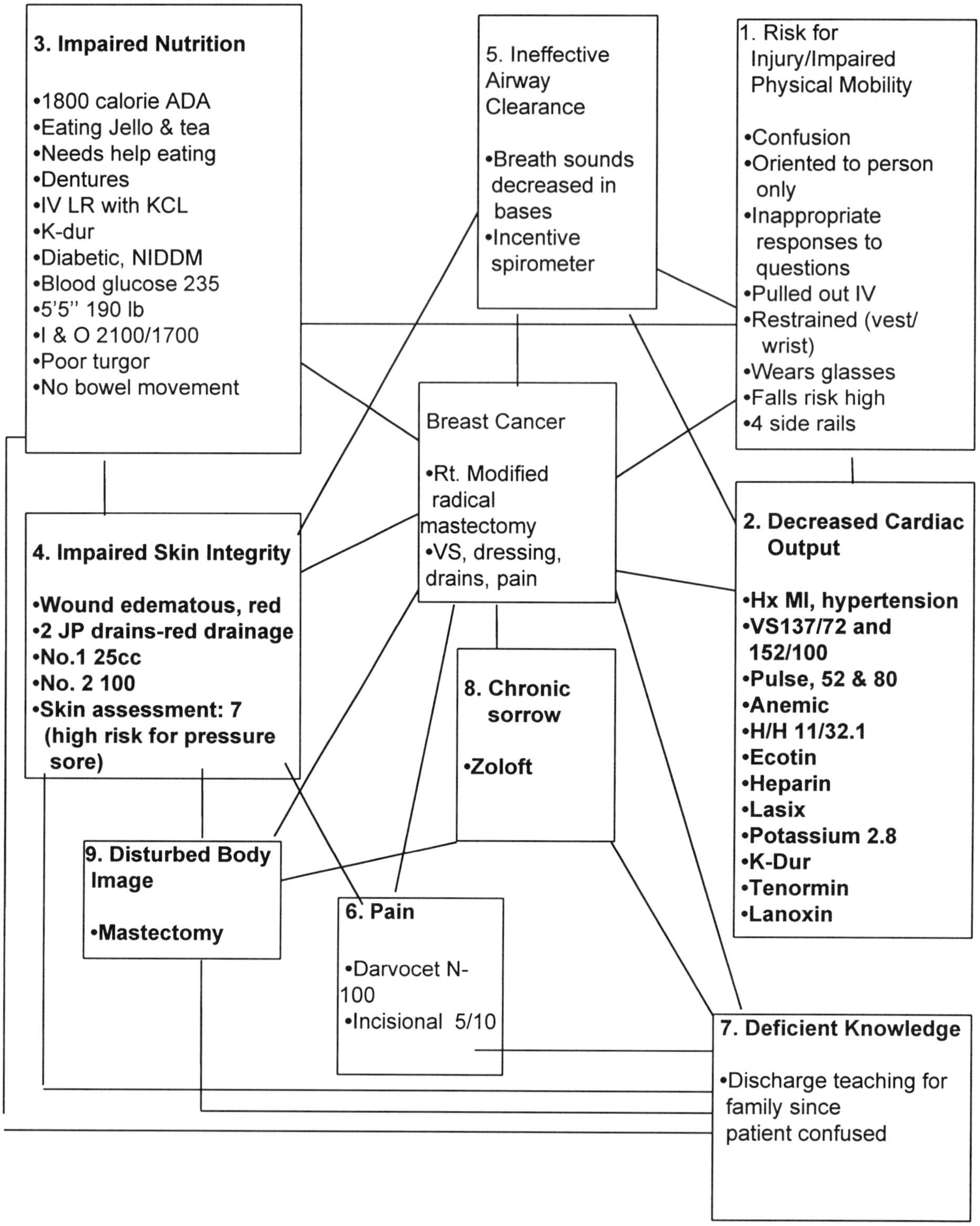
3. Impaired Nutrition
•1800 calorie ADA
•Eating Jello & tea
•Needs help eating
•Dentures
•IV LR with KCL
•K-dur
•Diabetic, NIDDM
•Blood glucose 235
•5'5" 190 lb
•I & O 2100/1700
•Poor turgor
•No bowel movement
5. Ineffective Airway Clearance
•Breath sounds decreased in bases
•Incentive spirometer
1. Risk for Injury/Impaired Physical Mobility
•Confusion
•Oriented to person only
•Inappropriate responses to questions
•Pulled out IV
•Restrained (vest/ wrist)
•Wears glasses
•Falls risk high
•4 side rails
Breast Cancer
•Rt. Modified radical mastectomy
•VS, dressing, drains, pain
4. Impaired Skin Integrity
•Wound edematous, red
•2 JP drains-red drainage
•No.1 25cc
•No. 2 100
•Skin assessment: 7 (high risk for pressure sore)
2. Decreased Cardiac Output
•Hx MI, hypertension
•VS137/72 and 152/100
•Pulse, 52 & 80
•Anemic
•H/H 11/32.1
•Ecotin
•Heparin
•Lasix
•Potassium 2.8
•K-Dur
•Tenormin
•Lanoxin
8. Chronic sorrow
•Zoloft
9. Disturbed Body Image
•Mastectomy
6. Pain
•Darvocet N-100
•Incisional 5/10
7. Deficient Knowledge
•Discharge teaching for family since patient confused

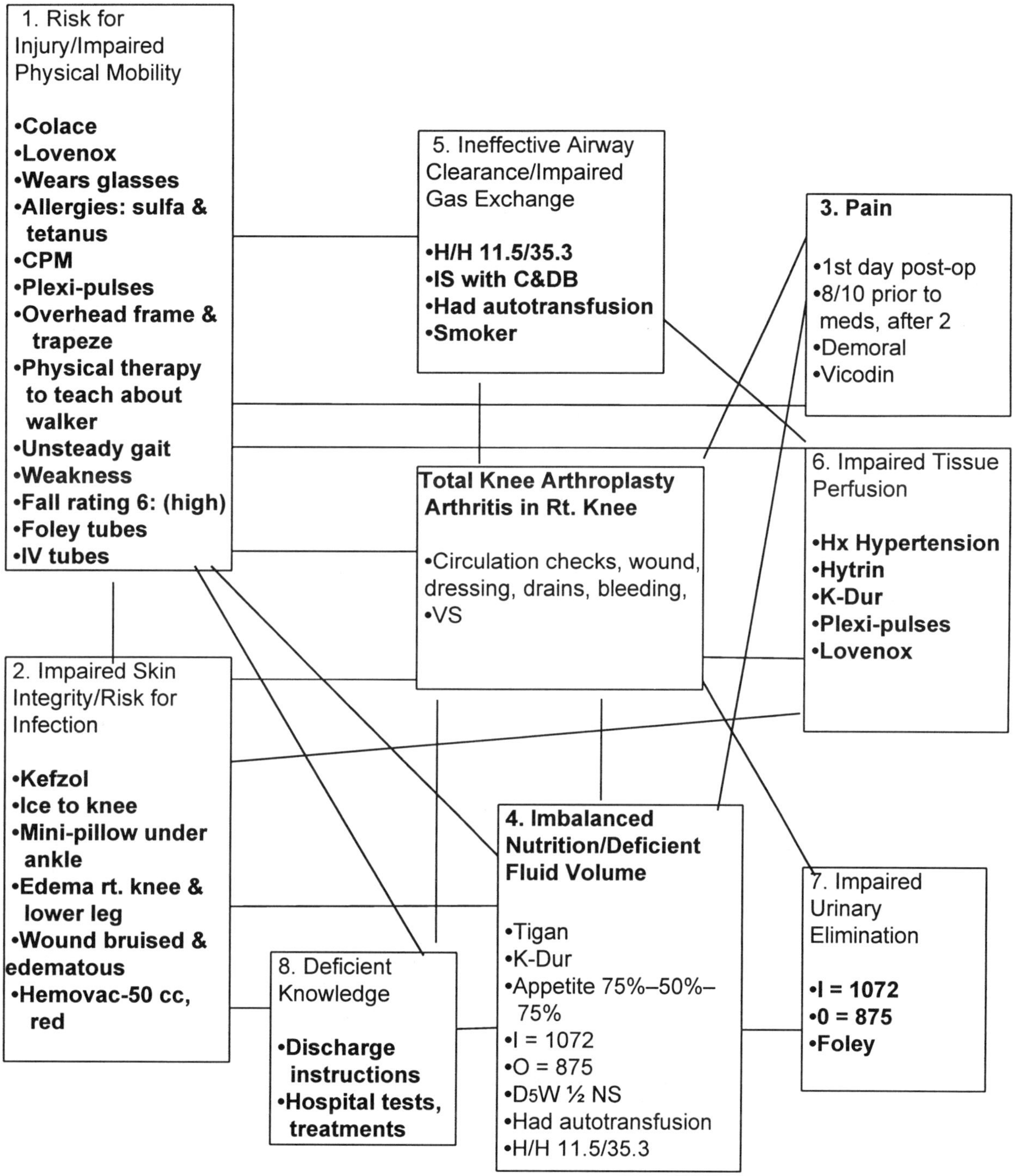
1. Risk for Injury/Impaired Physical Mobility
•Colace
•Lovenox
•Wears glasses
•Allergies: sulfa & tetanus
•CPM
•Plexi-pulses
•Overhead frame & trapeze
•Physical therapy to teach about walker
•Unsteady gait
•Weakness
•Fall rating 6: (high)
•Foley tubes
•IV tubes
5. Ineffective Airway Clearance/Impaired Gas Exchange
•H/H 11.5/35.3
•IS with C&DB
•Had autotransfusion
•Smoker
3. Pain
•1st day post-op
•8/10 prior to meds, after 2
•Demoral
•Vicodin
6. Impaired Tissue Perfusion
•Hx Hypertension
•Hytrin
•K-Dur
•Plexi-pulses
•Lovenox
Total Knee Arthroplasty Arthritis in Rt. Knee
•Circulation checks, wound, dressing, drains, bleeding,
•VS
2. Impaired Skin Integrity/Risk for Infection
•Kefzol
•Ice to knee
•Mini-pillow under ankle
•Edema rt. knee & lower leg
•Wound bruised & edematous
•Hemovac-50 cc, red
4. Imbalanced Nutrition/Deficient Fluid Volume
•Tigan
•K-Dur
•Appetite 75%–50%–75%
•I = 1072
•O = 875
•D5W ½ NS
•Had autotransfusion
•H/H 11.5/35.3
7. Impaired Urinary Elimination
•I = 1072
•0 = 875
•Foley
8. Deficient Knowledge
•Discharge instructions
•Hospital tests, treatments

Chapter 4

Nursing Interventions: So Many Problems, So Little Time

Writing goals, outcomes, and interventions is the last thing that has to be done before implementing nursing care. This reflects standards 3 and 4 of the American Nurses Association standards of clinical nursing practice. This chapter focuses on helping students learn to plan realistic and individualized goals, outcomes, and nursing interventions for each nursing diagnosis. Students must learn to incorporate both physical and psychosocial interventions in each plan of care. They have a tendency to focus on physical needs, with a minimal amount of attention to the psychosocial aspects of care. This will be addressed in detail in Chapter 6.

Because patient education is a central nursing role in many situations, a teaching plan needs to be developed for each patient and family. This chapter focuses on basic principles of patient teaching and learning, and on developing a one-page teaching plan. The one-page plan serves as a guide to patient and family teaching in clinical situations.

To effectively develop goals, outcomes, and interventions for the basic concept map care plan and the teaching plan, students need to learn how to use standardized care plan information. They must incorporate information in Step 4 from standardized care plans to be sure they have not missed any important aspects of the patient's care. Many faculty advocate using nursing interventions classifications (NIC)and nursing outcome classification (NOC) outcomes. Others recommend other standardized care plan guides as references for developing goals, outcomes, and interventions. Standardized care plans and teaching materials are available in many facilities and should be collected and used by students to develop and implement plans of care. Students need to be able to locate and use standardized nursing care plans, critical pathways, standard agency procedures, and patient education materials that apply to their patients. Students should be able to identify where patients are located on critical pathways, typical nursing care plans, and relevant patient teaching activities specific to the day they provide care. This activity implies they need to focus on outcomes for the specific day of care. Determining realistic outcomes for the day of care is a difficult task for many students.

Teaching Tips

It's important to guide students through the development of goals, outcomes, and objectives in a classroom setting. It is beneficial to have all students and clinical faculty in the room at the same time, so that everyone involved in teaching and learning this new process of concept map care planning has the same basic understanding. There will be course-specific goals, outcomes, and objectives to focus on. For example, in foundation courses, the focus will be on an individualized care plan for patients with safety, mobility, and skin integrity problems. In medical-surgical courses, the focus is on patient care concepts such as fluid balance, tissue perfusion, cardiac output, and gas exchange.

After completing class learning activities, be sure to summarize what all students need to bring with them to any clinical agency. I used to state this list verbally to students, but I've learned that a written checklist can be very beneficial in helping students to remember and get organized. It could include the following items:

1. Patient profile database. Use the database provided in Chapter 2 of this book or one that you have developed specific to your course.

2. Concept map based on the patient profile database (Steps 1 to 3). Use the forms provided in Chapter 1 of this book.

3. Plan of goals, outcomes, interventions (Step 4). Use the forms provided in Chapter 1 of this book.

4. Pressure ulcer and falls risk assessments. Use the forms from Chapter 3 of the student book or a standard agency form.

5. One-page teaching plan and patient education materials. Use the METHOD outline from Chapter 4 and collected education materials from the health-care agency.

6. Standardized care plans and critical pathways. Use those from the standardized care plan book or the health-care agency.

7. Medication cards or printouts of patient-specific medication information to support a discussion with faculty before administration.

Activity 1. Rationales and Sample Answers

Students should be assigned to work in groups of three or four to develop goals, outcomes, and interventions for scenarios 1 or 2. You may want to do one in class and the other as an assignment. Working in a group is beneficial for brainstorming ideas about care planning. Give each group one diagnosis from a scenario. Give them 15 minutes or so to come up with a plan for their assigned problem. Then have each group write the problem and their plan on the board. If you have enough room on the board, have students write the diagnoses at the same time so that all problems and plans are displayed simultaneously. Sample potential care plans are provided here as classroom guides. Your class may come up with variations in these plans, but as long as the major goals, outcomes, and interventions are included somewhere on the plan, that is what is important.

The Patient with Mastectomy

This is the more complex of the two sample plans because, in addition to the mastectomy, the patient is confused. Note that I have combined risk for injury, mobility, and confusion in Problem No. 1. You may prefer to separate them. But again, the idea is that all goals, outcomes, and interventions are included somewhere on the plan.

Problem No. 1: Risk for Injury, Impaired Physical Mobility, Acute Confusion **Goals:** Remains safe from injury, increased mobility, less confusion	
Outcomes: The patient will not be injured by falls or restraints, will move and cooperate, will not show signs of anxiety, will have improved orientation to place and time on the day of care.	
Nursing safety interventions, prevention of complications of immobility, reorient	Patient responses (will be done in the clinical setting)
1. Assess LOC, neurological signs q2h.	1.
2. Check restraints q1h.	2.
3. Maintain body in alignment.	3.
4. Change positions q2h.	4.
5. Perform ordered activity as tolerated—get up in chair for meals.	5.
6. Perform ROM exercises q2h.	6.
7. Have 4 siderails up while patient is in bed.	7.
8. Orient to day, hour, and location.	8.
9. Orient to reality—personal objects, clocks, calendars.	9.
10. Put glasses on patient while he/she is awake.	10.
11. Use empathy.	11.
12. Use distraction (TV, music, conversation).	12.
13. Use anticipatory guidance.	13.
14. Use reminiscence.	14.
15. Use comfort touches.	15.

Problem No. 2: Decreased Cardiac Output **Goals:** Improved cardiac output	
Outcomes: The patient will have stable vital signs, diastolic BP below 90, pulse above 60, and will cooperate in taking medications and drawing blood samples on the day of care.	
Nursing cardiac output interventions	Patient responses
1. Monitor VS q4h, with apical pulse.	1.
2. Check BP in left arm.	2.
3. Assess heart and chest pain.	3.
4. Assess extremities for edema and pulses.	4.
5. Have patient get up slowly to prevent orthostatic hypotension.	5.
6. Monitor laboratory reports H/H, K.	6.
7. Check about obtaining digitalis levels and blood coagulation studies.	7.
8. Administer medication.	8.

Problem No. 3: Impaired Nutrition, Feeding, Self-Care Deficit **Goals:** Improved nutrition	
Outcomes: The patient will eat 50% of all meals on the day of care.	
Nursing nutrition interventions	Patient responses (will be done in the clinical setting)
1. Assess GI system.	1.
2. Assess for BMs and GI upset.	2.
3. Assess intake and output.	3.
4. Monitor hydration: skin turgor, mucous membranes.	4.
5. Monitor appetite.	5.
6. Monitor IV fluids and site.	6.
7. Monitor blood glucose.	7.
8. Check about drug to control blood glucose.	8.
9. Have patient sit up in chair for meals.	9.
10. Clean and put in dentures.	10.
11. Assist with feedings as needed.	11.

Problem No. 4: Impaired Skin Integrity, Hygiene and Toileting Self-Care Deficits
Goals: Prevent infection, Skin remains intact (other than wound site)

Outcomes: The patient will have no signs or symptoms of wound infection and no signs of pressure ulcer development on day of care. Skin (other than wound site) is clean, dry, and intact all day.

Nursing skin integrity interventions	Patient responses
1. Assess wound site.	1.
2. Assess drain site.	2.
3. Assess amount and type of drainage JP No.1.	3.
4. Assess amount and type of drainage JP No.2.	4.
5. Monitor for arm edema and perform circulation checks.	5.
6. Monitor white blood cell count and temperature.	6.
7. Keep dressing dry and intact at all times.	7.
8. Perform sterile dressing change.	8.
9. Assist with bathing and hygiene, use moisturizers to prevent skin breakdown.	9.
10. Assist with toileting to prevent skin breakdown.	10.
11. Move patient carefully in bed to prevent sheering.	11.
(Nutrition: See problem No.3)	

(Mobility: See problem No.1)

Problem No. 5: Ineffective Airway Clearance
Goals: Improved breathing

Outcomes: The patient will use incentive spirometer q2h while awake, lung sounds remain clear for the day of care.

Nursing airway clearance interventions	Patient responses (will be done in the clinical setting)
1. Assess lungs, SOB.	1.
2. Use incentive spirometer q2h.	2.
3. Perform coughing and deep breathing q2h.	3.
4. Change positions; perform ROM as noted in Problem No. 1.	4.

Problem No. 6: Pain
Goals: Minimal Pain

Outcomes: The patient will report that pain is controlled and is less than 2 on a 10-point scale. Patient accepts pain medications if needed, performs exercises to decrease pain, accepts back massage, states feels comfortable.

Nursing pain interventions	Patient responses
1. Assess pain of incision using 10-point scale.	1.
2. Assess general comfort, ability to sleep.	2.
3. Do back massage with bath.	3.
4. Administer medications.	4.
5. Ensure warmth.	5.
6. Keep dressings clean and dry.	6.
7. Perform hygiene measures.	7.
8. Guide patient to do visual imagery, and perform relaxation techniques.	8.
9. Use comfort touch, hold hand.	9.
10. Look for nonverbal indicators of pain, such as restlessness and facial grimacing.	10.

Problem No. 7: Disturbed Body Image
Goals: Improve body image

Outcomes: The patient/family expresses thoughts and feelings, fixes patient's hair and makeup, and dresses patient in own clothes the day of care. Talks to inpatient women's health coordinator.

Nursing Body Image Interventions	Patient Responses
1. Actively listen and show empathy to encourage expression of thoughts and feelings concerning loss of breast (may not be applicable due to confusion).	1.
2. Help patient fix her hair and makeup.	2.
3. Get patient dressed in her own clothes.	3.
4. Collaborate with the inpatient women's health coordinator—a nurse who works with mastectomy patients.	4.
5. Refer patients and family to community resources for mastectomy patients.	5.

Problem No. 8: Deficient Knowledge
Goals: Improved knowledge of (family) since patient is confused. See teaching plan.

Problem No. 9: Chronic Sorrow. This diagnosis may be premature. We need to do further patient assessment. Zoloft is an antidepressant, but there is no assessment data to indicate the reason for the prescription. The psychosocial assessment in Chapter 6 would be helpful in determining the need for the drug.

The patient with a knee replacement

This sample scenario Step 4 of care planning may make the best take home assignment because it is not as complex as the previous example.

Problem No. 1: Risk for Injury, Impaired Physical Mobility **Goals:** Remains safe from injury, increased mobility	
Outcomes: The patient will not be injured by falls, will use CPM, and correctly use walker to assist with walking on the day of care.	
Nursing safety interventions, Prevention of complications of immobility	Patient responses (will be done in the clinical setting)
1. Maintain body in alignment.	1.
2. Reinforce need for WBAT (to prevent dislocation).	2.
3. Keep mini-pillow under ankle.	3.
4. Change positions q2h.	4.
5. Help patient sit up in chair for meals.	5.
6. Assess gait and weakness.	6.
7. Perform ROM exercises q2h.	7.
8. CPM for 3 hours after lunch.	8.
9. Keep two siderails up while in bed.	9.
10. Use plexi-pulses while in bed.	10.
11. Administer medications.	11.
12. Tell patient to wear glasses while awake.	12.
13. Have patient use trapeze to pull himself up.	13.
14. Have patient use walker for ambulation.	14.
15. Check that PT teaches patient about walker.	15.

16. Get help from two other students when getting him up for the first time.	16.
17. Be careful of tubes when getting him up.	17.
18. Check for orthostatic hypotension, and get patient up slowly.	18.

Problem No. 2: Impaired Skin Integrity **Goals:** Prevent infection, Skin remains intact (other than wound site)
Outcomes: The patient will have no signs or symptoms of wound infection, no signs of pressure ulcer development on day of care. Skin (other than wound site) is clean, dry, and intact all day.

Nursing skin integrity interventions	Patient responses
1. Assess wound site.	1.
2. Apply ice pack to knee.	2.
3. Assess drain site.	3.
4. Assess amount and type of drainage from Hemovac.	4.
5. Monitor for leg for edema, check circulation.	5.
6. Keep mini-pillow under ankle.	6.
7. Monitor white blood cell count and temperature.	7.
8. Keep dressing dry and intact at all times.	8.
9. Perform sterile dressing change.	9.
10. Assist with bathing and hygiene to avoid skin breakdown.	10.
11. Use lotions and massage after bathing.	11.
12. Assist with toileting to prevent skin breakdown.	12.
13. Use trapeze to prevent sheering.	13.
14. Administer medications.	14.

(Nutrition. See problem No. 4)

(Mobility. See problem No. 1)

Problem No. 3: Pain
Goals: Minimal pain

Outcomes: The patient will report that pain is controlled and is less than 2 on a 10-point scale, accepts pain medications if needed, performs techniques to decrease pain, accepts back massage, and states feels comfortable.

Nursing pain interventions	Patient responses
1. Assess pain of incision using 10-point scale.	1.
2. Assess general comfort and ability to sleep.	2.
3. Do back massage with bath.	3.
4. Administer medications.	4.
5. Ensure warmth.	5.
6. Keep dressings clean and dry.	6.
7. Perform hygiene measures.	7.
8. Guide patient to do visual imagery, relaxation techniques.	8.
9. Monitor for chest pain (emboli) and SOB.	9.
10. Monitor for severe joint pain (displacement).	10.

Problem No. 4: Impaired Nutrition/Deficient Fluid Volume **Goals:** Improved nutrition & fluid volume	
Outcomes: The patient will eat 75% of all meals on the day of care.	
Nursing nutrition interventions	Patient responses (will be done in the clinical setting)
1. Assessment GI system.	1.
2. Assess for BMs, GI upset, and nausea.	2.
3. Assess intake and output.	3.
4. Monitor K; check to see last K level.	4.
5. Administer K-Dur.	5.
6. Monitor hydration (skin turgor, mucous membranes).	6.
7. Monitor appetite.	7.
8. Monitor IV fluids and site.	8.
9. Monitor H/H.	9.
10. Have patient sit up in chair for meals.	10.
11. Medicate for nausea if needed.	11.

Problem No. 5: Ineffective Airway Clearance
Goals: Improved breathing

Outcomes: The patient will use incentive spirometer q2h while awake, lung sounds remain clear for the day of care.

Nursing airway clearance interventions	Patient responses (will be done in the clinical setting)
1. Assess lungs, SOB.	1.
2. Use incentive spirometer q2h.	2.
3. Have patient perform coughing and deep breathing q2h.	3.
4. Perform position changes, ROM as noted in Problem No. 1.	4.
5. Assess interest in quitting smoking.	5.
6. Remind patient of hospital smoking policies.	6.

Problem No. 6: Impaired Tissue Perfusion
Goals: Improve tissue perfusion

Outcomes: The patient's blood pressure will be less than 140/90 the day of care.

Nursing tissue perfusion interventions	Patient responses
1. Monitor VS q4h.	1.
2. Administer medications.	2.
3. Use plexi-pulses while in bed.	3.
4. Get patient up slowly to prevent orthostatic hypotension.	4.

(See immobility No. 1.)

(See skin integrity No. 2.)

Problem No. 7: Impaired Urinary Elimination
Goals: Improve urinary elimination

Outcomes: The patient's has no signs or symptoms of UTI, and intake approximately equals output, although outputs may be less than input first 48 hours post-op.

Nursing elimination interventions	Patient responses
1. Assess S/S of UTI.	1.
2. Monitor intake.	2.
3. Monitor output.	3.
4. Monitor patency of Foley catheter.	4.

Problem No. 8: Deficient Knowledge regarding discharge planning, hospital routines. See teaching plan.

Activity 2. Rationales and Sample Answers

General rationales are given for interventions with each of the listed problems in the scenarios.

The Patient with Mastectomy

Problem 1

Ongoing assessment of neurological status is very important for this patient because she is confused and restrained. The patient needs to be re-oriented to day, hour, location, personal objects, and familiar people to help attain this objective. She will need her glasses to see her surroundings. Restraints and siderails are required to keep the patient safe from injury and falls. Restraints must be checked frequently to ensure adequate circulation in the extremities and to be sure the patient's body remains in correct alignment. Psychologically supportive interventions are important to calm a patient who is confused; these include use of comforting touches, empathy, and distraction. The patient may be able to reminisce and talk about her past life, which may serve as a distraction and meet growth and developmental needs. Anticipatory guidance and touch are needed to support all treatments and ensure the patient's cooperation. Getting the patient up and moving and doing range-of-motion (ROM) activities avoids problems associated with immobility. Positions must be changed frequently, and the patient should be sitting up for breakfast and lunch and should even go for a walk if able.

Problem 2

Ongoing assessment of cardiovascular status is important because of the patient's history of hypertension and myocardial infarction and recent increase in blood pressure and abnormally low pulse. Assessment of vital signs, apical pulse, edema, and pulses in the extremities is very important. Circulation on the operative side is important because of complications of lymphedema. Also, blood pressure should be taken and IVs placed on the unoperative arm to avoid complications of edema and infection when lymph nodes have been removed. The patient's K is very low, and the digitalis level is not known. The most current values need to be obtained because abnormal electrolyte balance and digitalis toxicity may be the cause of the confusion. In addition, the patient is taking an anticoagulant and aspirin and there is no information on blood coagulation, so this assessment is essential. Continue monitoring the H/H for blood loss postoperatively; the values are slightly low in this patient.

Problem 3

Nutritional problems require GI assessments and noting of bowel movements and upper GI distress such as belching or nausea. Checking hydration is part of the assessment for nutrition. Intake and output with anyone receiving an IV is important, and this patient has not been eating well. Making sure she uses her dentures, sitting her up to eat, and assisting her with feedings may improve intake. The blood glucose needs to be further assessed because the patient's blood glucose level is high enough to warrant a medication. She has a history of

NIDDM, so a key question is, why isn't she currently on a medication when her blood glucose is that high?

Problem 4

Interventions for skin integrity in surgical patients are centered on assessment, care of the wound, and monitoring of infection and bleeding. Checking for edema and circulation on the operative side is specific to the patient with mastectomy. In addition, this patient is at risk for skin breakdown and will need assistance with toileting, bathing, and hygiene because of her confusion. She must be moved up in bed carefully to prevent sheering of skin. Poor nutrition and immobility contribute to skin breakdown.

Problem 5

Interventions to improve airway clearance and prevent complications such as pneumonia are needed in all surgical patients. Routine prevention in surgical patients includes the using an incentive spirometer, prescribing coughing and deep breathing exercises, and getting the patient up and moving as quickly as possible. Immobility was covered in Problem No. 1.

Problem 6

Pain is another problem common to surgical patients. Students need to note all pharmacologic and nonpharmacologic methods of pain control. In this patient, basic hygiene and warmth are key considerations, and comfort touches would be used to decrease anxiety. Anxiety and lack of comfort increase pain. The student could also attempt to do visual imagery or relaxation techniques, but these may not be realistic with a confused patient. Patients who are confused may not communicate their discomfort. Assess general comfort and nonverbal pain indicators such as restlessness, grimacing, and inability to sleep.

Problem 7

It may be assumed that the patient has an altered body image because of the mastectomy. Patients need to be able to express thoughts and feelings, and a primary communication technique to use is empathy to help patients express emotions. This may not be possible because the patient is confused. However, the nurse could help to improve her body image by making the patient look and feel as good as possible by assisting with basic hygienic practices such as bathing, fixing her hair, and helping with makeup if she usually wears it. She should also be dressed in her own nightgowns because they look better than hospital gowns. Students should be aware of hospital-based health educators and community resources to assist patients with emotional and physical changes that occur with chronic illnesses such as cancer and, in this case, mastectomy.

Problem 8

A teaching plan for deficient knowledge is included in Activity 3. Teaching is not possible with a confused patient, so the plan would be implemented with the family, if they are available. Always the first thing to do is to assess current knowledge and interests, and then to proceed with topics based on patient and family interests. Urge students to follow principles of adult learning and to make connections with agency health educators and community resources.

Problem 9

The diagnosis of chronic sorrow is premature. Further assessment regarding the reason for taking the drug is needed. The plan simply involves further assessment before developing a more specific plan.

The Patient with a Knee Replacement

Problem 1

Preventing complications of immobility and injury is essential in the patient with musculoskeletal surgeries and disease. Assessment of gait and weakness is required, and the patient's activity is "weight bearing as tolerated." Emphasize that extreme care is needed in getting the patient up, especially for the first time. Patients with glasses should always wear them to avoid falls. The IV and the Foley catheter are also potential fall risks. There is also a potential for orthostatic hypotension in all surgical patients from blood loss and pain medications. This patient must remain in proper alignment to avoid dislocating the knee, so remind students to position him properly using pillows.

Physical therapists are involved in teaching patients exercises and use of the walker for ambulation, and nurses would reinforce those initial instructions and also make sure the patient is using the walker properly. Return of function to the leg is facilitated and prevention of complications of immobility by position changes is enhanced. Use of the trapeze facilitates changing positions. Use of the CPM, range-of-motion (ROM), and muscle-strengthening exercises is required to regain function quickly. The plexi-pulses and Lovenox prevent formation of blood clots in the extremities, a serious complication of immobility. Colace is to prevent constipation, a complication of immobility.

Problem 2

Skin integrity rationales are the same as for the mastectomy patient. Note that this patient also has an ice pack to decrease swelling. He also has a prophylactic antibiotic added to the regimen to prevent infection.

Problem 3

Pain interventions and rationales are similar to those for the patient with mastectomy. However, it will be necessary to monitor the patient for chest pain due to pulmonary emboli, a serious complication of this type of surgery and immobility. Also, be aware that severe pain in the joint could indicate displacement or hemorrhage.

Problem 4

Nutritional intervention rationales are the same as those for the mastectomy patient. The patient has a medication added for nausea in case it is needed. Potassium should be monitored in anyone receiving supplements. Hemoglobin and hematocrit are essential in this patient with his history of autotransfusion and the possibility of continued bleeding in a joint after this type of surgery.

Problem 5

Promoting adequate ventilation and preventing complications is essential in all surgical patients, so rationales are similar to those for the mastectomy patient. However, this patient is a smoker and is therefore at increased risk for respiratory complications. If the patient is interested in quitting, referrals may be made to community resources, and he may receive medications to assist in smoking cessation. Hospital smoking policies must be followed to ensure fire safety precautions.

Problem 6

The patient is on an antihypertensive drug and must have special attention paid to his vital signs. Orthostatic hypotension is possible in any surgical patient, especially those with blood loss who are on narcotics. Plexi-pulses improve circulation while in bed.

Problem 7

Urinary elimination is managed with a Foley catheter in some surgical patients to monitor output. Catheter patency must be monitored along with its primary complication; that is, urinary tract infection.

Problem 8

Develop a teaching plan. Before teaching anything, students should always determine the patient's current knowledge and motivation and should follow principles of adult learning. They should make connections between agency educators and the patient/family, and make referrals to community resources after discharge as applicable to the patient's needs.

Activity 3.

An outline of the METHOD teaching plan appears on the next page, followed by formatted teaching plans for a patient with a knee replacement and a patient with a mastectomy and confusion.

METHOD Daily Teaching Plan

Patient Name:

Diagnosis:

Teaching Techniques:

M (Medications):

E (Environment):

T (Treatments):

H (Health Knowledge of Disease):

O (Outpatient/Inpatient Referrals):

D (Diet):

Source: P. Schuster: Communication: The Key to the Therapeutic Relationship, FA Davis, 2000.

Teaching Plan: Patient with a Knee Replacement

This teaching plan would primarily involve teaching regarding self-care at home but would also include information on inpatient drugs, treatments and procedures as needed.

Medications

K-Dur—potassium supplement, twice a day

Hytrin—for blood pressure, one a day

Colace—a stool softener to prevent constipation, once a day

Lovenox—to prevent formation of blood clots (injection at home)

Demoral—for severe pain (in hospital only)

Vicodin—for moderate pain (may go home with this)

Tigan—for nausea (in hospital only)

Environment

Assess whether the patient's wife or other family members will help the patient with self-care and provide transportation after discharge. A home–health-care visit should be scheduled to explain safety in the home and assist with self-care. Physical therapy will continue at home. Teaching booklets can help explain home safety measures, such as removing scatter rugs, installing grab bars at tub and toilet, maintaining adequate lighting, and so on.

Treatments

Demonstrate use of walker. Demonstrate isometric exercises. Demonstrate Lovenox injection. Describe wound care procedures. Demonstrate proper application and monitoring of CPM machine. Demonstrate use of incentive spirometer.

Health Knowledge of Disease

Describe signs and symptoms of infection of the wound, and explain the need for each treatment listed above. The patient should know which activities are allowed and which positions should be maintained or avoided (no flexion of greater than 90 degrees).

Outpatient/Inpatient Referrals

The patient should know when to schedule a physician outpatient visit and that visiting home-care nurses and physical therapists are scheduled to come to his home.

Diet

The patient may eat a regular diet. Emphasize the need for protein and vitamin C to aid wound healing and fiber to prevent constipation. The patient should receive a copy of the food pyramid from Chapter 2 to use as a guide for healthy meal planning.

Teaching Plan: Patient with Mastectomy and Confusion

The teaching that needs to be done concerns the plans of care in the inpatient setting. The teaching would be done with the family because the patient is confused.

Medications

Give the reason for each medication (if asked).

Heparin—thins blood to prevent complications of immobility after surgery

Lasix—a diuretic to remove excess fluids from the body

Tenormin—to control blood pressure

K-Dur—to replace potassium loss from the diuretic

Zoloft—an antidepressant (Tell students that they may want to ask family members if they know the reason for this drug.)

Lanoxin—to improve heart function

Ecotin—aspirin to prevent further heart attacks

Darvocet N-100—for control of pain

Environment

Tell students to be prepared to give the reason for restraints and what is being done to re-orient the patient. Tell the family to talk to the patient about things that interest her and to hold her hand. Family members can be useful in re-orienting patients and encouraging them to cooperate.

Treatments

Explain the need for the dressing change, and give information that the wound is healing as expected (provided it is). Emphasize to students the need to explain the incentive spirometer to family members and to encourage family members to help the patient use it.

Health Knowledge of Disease

It is currently unknown why the patient is confused. Family members will need reassurance that tests are being done to find out. Patient and families will want to know the outcomes of biopsies. The physician will inform them, but the nurse may need to reiterate after the physician gives initial information.

Outpatient/inpatient Referrals

Explain the role of the women's health coordinator and reasons for blood work, such as potassium, glucose, and digitalis levels.

Diet

The patient is on an 1800-calorie ADA diet. If the family and patient desire, they may assist with helping her to eat. Explain the need for protein and vitamin C to heal wounds.

Activity 4.

Teaching methods and evaluation techniques should be used in implementing the teaching plan of care. Teaching methods and evaluation techniques include the following:

Cognitive knowledge is taught giving explanations and descriptions, and using books, pamphlets, films, programmed instruction, or computer programs. It is evaluated with oral or written questions, or having the patient keep a diary or written record for self-monitoring.

Affective knowledge (and cognitive knowledge) is gained by using one-on-one discussion, group discussion, role playing, or discovery to guide the patient to problem-solve situations that may be encountered. The patient can express feelings and use cognitive knowledge to solve problems. Affective knowledge is evaluated by inferring how the patient responds, speaks, or verbally expresses feelings and values.

Psychomotor knowledge is taught by using demonstrations accompanied by explanations. Psychomotor knowledge is evaluated by a return demonstration.

Activity 5.

This activity gives the students practice in developing psychosocial interventions that can be used in a variety of clinical situations. Anxiety is a common emotion in many patients and needs to be assessed. Key interventions to decrease anxiety include empathy, therapeutic touch, and humor.

Anxiety Assessment

I would ask the patient: What's wrong? What's going on? What's happening?

I would look for verbal and nonverbal behaviors that indicate anxiety:

Sample Nonverbal: Restlessness, poor eye contact, trembling, inability to concentrate, facial tension, flushing, voice quivering, increased wariness, irritability, increased perspiration, sweaty palms, foot shuffling, arm movements, or increased blood pressure and pulse.

Sample Verbal: Stating feelings of being jittery, distressed, or dizzy; crying; or direct expression of concerns. Anxiety may cause reports of physical discomforts such as GI discomforts, headache, backache, palpitations, or dry mouth.

Empathy

In anxious patients, students should use empathy to help them express their concerns. Urge them to use verbal and nonverbal behaviors by saying something like, "I see you are restless (trembling, etc). What's wrong? Are you nervous about something?" They also can use nonverbal active listening skills and sit down with the patient if possible.

Caring Touch

Anxious patients may respond to hand holding or touching a shoulder. The touches can be used in conjunction with communication techniques such as empathy and active listening.

Humor

Humor can sometimes be used to reduce mild anxiety and facilitate establishing a therapeutic relationship. They student could joke about the food, for example, "I bet we're having filet mignon for lunch today. What do you think?" Remind students that they can use humor to establish an open exchange with the patient, but that they should get serious if the patient expresses concerns or worries.

Chapter 5

Using Concept Map Care Plans in the Health-care Agency

Students need to learn organizational strategies for successful clinical performance. This can be accomplished with concept map care plans. This chapter focuses on using concept maps in outpatient and inpatient clinical settings, and particularly on implementation and evaluation of clinical care based on standard 5 of the American Nurses Association Standards of clinical practice.

The concept map care plan is used as a clinical organizational tool and is updated and revised throughout the clinical day to guide practice and evaluation. It facilitates communication between students, clinical faculty, and agency staff nurses. A special benefit of using concept map care plans includes guiding students to identify relationships between medications and relevant clinical data, such as laboratory test reports and signs and symptoms of disease.

Students often have difficulty identifying patient responses, especially those that are psychological or sociological responses. Step 5 of the concept map care plan is specifically designed to focus students on patient responses. Students carry the maps into patient rooms as they interact with patients, and they evaluate patient responses to nursing interventions as they proceed throughout the clinical day.

Teaching Tips

If the basic concept map care plan with the teaching plan has been prepared the night before clinical, then students will need to get organized on arrival to the inpatient setting the next day. Students need help in getting organized. I recommend giving students a written "To Do" list, with an explanation of why each item on the list is important. A written checklist is beneficial to foundations students because it helps remind them what they are to do. Review the following sequence of activities and how to use the concept map to take notes and organize activities. Each of the items on this list is covered in the chapter but needs to be verbally emphasized. Becuase concept care map plans are modified throughout the clinical day, you'll need to tell students to use a contrasting color of ink, such as red. As you make revisions and add to the concept map care plans, use a third color of ink, such as purple or green.

"To Do" List on Arrival to the Inpatient Setting

1. Check medication record.

Students should note specific times of administration and dosages that may have changed, or new medication orders. Medication orders change at a rapid rate in the inpatient setting, and students must keep themselves up to date. Because correctly administering medications requires extreme caution to avoid errors, medications should be highlighted on map diagrams. Highlighting is done so that medications stand out.

2. Check IV record.

Students should note the rates of infusion, when the IV is due to be changed, and the times of administration if the IV is intermittent. They should highlight IVs on the concept map diagrams so that they stand out.

3. Check treatments.

Have students write updates on map diagrams and Step 4, if needed, noting times a treatment is supposed to be done.

4. Obtain report from off-going shift.

Have students write updates on map diagrams and Step 4 if needed.

5. Check concept maps preconference.

Students should use concept map care plans to give you priority information about their patient. You can glance at the concept map care plans and see if students have accurately analyzed data, identified realistic outcomes, and identified appropriate ongoing nursing assessments and interventions. Of course, that does not guarantee students will follow through and do what they wrote, but at least you and other faculty are aware of whether students have the cognitive knowledge required to implement care. This is one of the best aspects of concept map care plans: Faculty can see a comprehensive plan before clinical. Concept map care plans were devised to avoid student and faculty frustration in preconferences because students were not well prepared for patient care. After using concept map care plans, many faculty have reported that preconferences go very smoothly.

6. Complete key assessments.

Students should put the maps in their pockets and then go and do the assessments they have identified as "key assessments" in the center box on the concept map diagram. Key assessments are one aspect of Step 2 of the concept map care plan. Students record key assessments after they have completed them, Step 5 of the concept map care plan. Patient responses are numbered to correspond to nursing assessment interventions that were identified in Step 4. The interventions and responses are directly linked. This is because interventions

(Step 4) and responses (Step 5) are listed across from each other and are numbered the same way on the concept map care plan.

7. Find RN cover, introduce yourself, and report abnormalities.

Tell students to use their concept map care plans to give a report on abnormalities in assessment data. They should write whatever the nurse tells them on the concept map care plan if it is not already specified in the plan of care. Many students need to learn to be assertive and tactful as they interrupt a busy staff nurse.

8. Find faculty and report abnormalities.

Jointly look at the concept map care plan as the student gives assessment updates. Check the student's modifications to the concept map care plan based on new data. Emphasize that you want to hear from each student even though you may be very busy.

9. Find medications.

Tell students to make sure all medications are on the unit and to get them if they are not available. They should know when a medication will be delivered or if someone needs to go get it. Students should use the medication administration record and the concept map care plan as they check for availability of medications.

10. Go to medication area 30 minutes before drug is needed.

Tell students to make sure they have obtained updated laboratory reports and assessment data needed to safely administer drugs. Use the concept map diagram as you discuss each drug with the student. This helps students to process information (think critically) and learn the important relationships between medications, laboratory data, and symptoms by seeing the information listed under specific problems they have identified on the concept map diagram.

Bedside Guides

Concept map care plans are bedside guides to care. Students check off interventions (Step 4) as they complete them, and they carefully watch for and record patient responses to interventions (Step 5). Students and faculty can discuss progress towards outcomes and goals as they go through the day. Faculty can make notations on concept map care plans as needed. Some faculty in critical care settings have told me that they tape maps to bedside stands, and the maps have become the focus of patient care discussions between nurses, physicians, and students.

Learning Activities: Rationales and Sample Answers

Activity 1

A valuable learning activity during preconference is for students with similar patients to compare concept map care plans. The purpose of this exercise is to find similarities in all patients with a particular reason for admission, and then to become cognizant of individual differences based on specifics of the assessment of unique patients.

Activity 2

After completion of Chapter 5, students are prepared to devise a plan of care and implement and evaluate it on a real patient assignment in an inpatient or outpatient setting.

Activity 3

Lecture Class Exercise: Students need to bring completed concept map care plans to class. Those assigned to patients with similar diagnoses should form groups and review patient responses. The purpose of this exercise is to compare Step 5 (patient responses) in patients with similar diagnoses. Students realize that although the patients may have similar problems and interventions, the verbal and nonverbal responses listed under Step 5 are unique, and progress towards outcomes varies.

Activity 4

Compare and contrast the concept map diagram developed for the diabetic inpatient scenario in Figure 5–2 and the concept map diagram for the outpatient undergoing endoscopy procedures in Figure 5–3. The point of this exercise is to compare inpatient and outpatient maps so that students recognize that outpatient maps are very general guides based on typical problems that occur in most patients in the outpatient setting. The diagram is a standardized diagram because there is no specific patient data until a patient assessment has been completed. Concept map diagrams based on real patient data are individualized and specific guides for individualized holistic nursing care.

Chapter 6

Mapping Psychosocial Problems

Mapping psychosocial problems is the focus of Chapter 6. Identification and management of psychosocial problems is often more difficult than the management of physical problems for many students. Students can use the Psychosocial Assessment Tool to guide them in recognizing problems as they interact with patients. Therapeutic communication techniques are the foundation of nursing practice and need to be integrated into every plan of care and used during each patient interaction. Emphasize to students that all concept map care plans must include psychosocial problems and therapeutic communication techniques.

I wrote a book about the essential aspects of therapeutic communication titled *Communication: The Key to the Therapeutic Relationship,* published by F.A. Davis in 2000. This communication book was written as an adjunct to concept map care plans.

It is designed especially for nursing foundations students and is focused on helping students learn how to communicate in "difficult" situations during the first days of clinical experience. I have referred to this book throughout Chapter 6. Students must recognize and respond to basic emotional reactions to health-care situations from the first day on a clinical unit to the very last day of their careers in nursing. Many students need to learn how to be more assertive, responsive, and self-confident. They need to become more aware of cultural differences and gender differences that affect the nature of human responses. Nursing psychosocial interventions are based on the assessment of gender differences, self-esteem, and body image, and on recognizing typical emotional patterns of behavior. During foundations courses, nurses need to learn the most basic communication interventions such as empathy, touch, and humor, and also what to do if the patient cries. They need to use therapeutic communication as they educate patients. In addition, they must learn how to use therapeutic communication to guide patients in identifying problems and then use the problem-solving process to guide patients and families in making decisions. These are fundamentals students must learn to assess so they can intervene in psychosocially stressful and difficult emotional situations.

Teaching Tips

Psychosocial assessments and recognition of problems are made throughout the clinical day. There is very little known from the data that is collected the night before clinical because there is not much time spent in interaction with the patient. If students get to meet the patient and introduce themselves, they may be able to determine the patient's basic emotional state. During interactions with patients, students should use the psychosocial assessment tool to focus on assessing and determining:

1. Current emotional state
2. Patient's life experiences regarding health care
3. Family's ability to cope and support the patient
4. Growth and development disruptions caused by health problems
5. Relations with health-care providers
6. Self-concept alterations: self-esteem and body image
7. Cultural conflicts
8. Gender issues

Most students can detect the patient's or family member's mood without difficulty; for example, whether the patient or family member is contented and happy, or anxious, fearful, sad, hopeless, lonely, angry, and so on. The key factors negatively impacting the emotional state include bad life experiences with health care leading up to the present situation, a family that is unable to cope and is nonsupportive, the inability to accomplish growth and developmental goals, dissatisfaction with health-care providers, poor self-concept, cultural conflicts, and gender differences in communication creating conflict.

As soon as the student recognizes an emotional/psychosocial problem, it should be put in a box on the concept map diagram with the evidence to support it. Then, you and the student can develop an "on-the-spot" goal, patient objectives, and interventions to be implemented immediately. A typical goal would be to increase the patient's ability to cope with the emotion. The patient objective would be for the patient to talk about what is creating the problem, and the key intervention in this situation is empathy.

Students need to know what empathy is and how to be empathic. They must be told to verbalize understanding of the emotion and then accept the emotion. Then they must listen and ask questions to identify the problem that is causing the emotion. Empathy is easy to define and explain but takes much practice to effectively use as a clinical communication intervention.

The objective of using empathy is to get patients to express concerns about perceived problems. Students must then assist patients with problem solving, so focus teaching on steps in the problem-solving process:

1. Identify a general problem (using empathy and listening skills).
2. Search out information. (Faculty serve as resources of information.)
3. Examine options.

4. Discuss pros and cons of each option.
5. Allow the patient and family to choose an option.
6. Develop a plan.
7. Implement a plan.
8. Evaluate if plan is effective.

Other therapeutic interventions to describe and discuss include:

Therapeutic humor: Health-care providers can joke, kid, clown, or mimic and laugh at imperfections in themselves and laugh with others about the imperfect nature of situations. Therapeutic humor should be distinguished from nontherapeutic humor.

Therapeutic response to crying: Health-care providers can encourage emotional release through tears and words and allow patients to regain control using silence and acceptance of response. Comforting touch and offering tissues may be appropriate. Students should also know what not to do when someone cries.

Therapeutic use of touch: Health-care providers can use caring touches such as placing an arm around the patient's shoulder, hugging or patting on the back, playful hitting or poking, or handholding during procedures or when patients cry. Caring touches should be distinguished from task touches and protective touches. The student should be aware of situations where touch is not appropriate.

Learning Activities: Rationales and Sample Answers

Activity 1

The purpose of this activity is for students to share clinical experiences in which they used communication techniques to establish therapeutic relationships with patients. They should give examples of empathy, humor, touch, what they did when the patient or family member cried, and examples of use of problem solving with patients. Other communication techniques include positive reinforcement, encouragement, distraction, reality orientation, reminiscing, anticipatory guidance, and showing positive regard. Discuss specific verbal and nonverbal responses to the techniques. Have students write examples on the board.

Activity 2

The purpose of this activity is to have students explore cultural backgrounds in themselves and classmates and to share similarities and differences. The Mini–Cultural Assessment Tool (see Fig. 6–6) could be completed as a take-home assignment to review with family members (friends or roommates) and then shared in small groups during class. Small groups are less threatening in which to share personal information. The groups can then summarize information in categories so that it is not personal when presented to the larger class.

Activity 3

After you have discussed the psychosocial assessment tool and students have had some time in clinical situations, use this activity to allow students to share clinical experiences that provide examples of assessment data that led to the determination that the patient had psychosocial problems. Students should give examples for each category of the psychosocial assessment tool including emotional state, the patient's life experiences, family, growth and development, relations with health-care providers, self-esteem, body image, culture, and gender issues. Have students write examples on the board.

Activity 4

The answers to the practice exercises for developing psychosocial nursing diagnoses with supporting verbal and nonverbal patient assessment data are below in bold. For each feeling, a psychosocial nursing diagnosis is to be written along with common verbal and nonverbal behaviors that are signs and symptoms of the emotion. The purpose of Activity No. 4 is for students to become familiar with psychosocial nursing diagnoses.

Anxious

Nursing Diagnosis: Anxiety—vague feeling of discomfort or dread from a nonspecific cause

Verbal: Quivering voice, expressed concerns, confusion

Nonverbal: Poor eye contact, restlessness, fidgeting, irritability, tremors, signs and symptoms of stress response ("fight or flight"—general adaptation syndrome)

Fearful

Nursing Diagnosis: Fear—anxiety caused by a perceived threat of recognized danger

Verbal: Identifies and states object of fear

Nonverbal: Frightened—symptoms of stress response—may become aggressive or withdraw, depending on usual response patterns

Sad

Nursing Diagnosis: Chronic Sorrow—pervasive sadness experienced in response to continual loss throughout the trajectory of an illness.

Verbal: Expresses wide range of emotions including sadness, anger, confusion, disappointment, emptiness, frustration, helplessness, hopelessness, loneliness

Nonverbal: Tears, withdrawal from situations, unwillingness to verbalize, aggressive gestures with anger

Hopeless

Nursing Diagnosis: Hopelessness—patient sees no choices in a situation and is unable to mobilize energy to overcome perceived obstacles.

Verbal: Verbalizes “I can’t…”

Nonverbal: Passive, decreased affect, closed eyes, decreased verbalizations, decreased responses to stimuli

Lonely

Nursing Diagnosis: Social Isolation—negative feelings experienced from being alone that are perceived as imposed by others

Verbal: Expressions of rejection

Nonverbal: Absence of supportive significant others

Out of control

Nursing Diagnosis: Powerlessness—perceived lack of control over a situation.

Verbal: Verbal expressions of lack of control

Nonverbal: Nonparticipation when opportunities are provided, reluctance to express feelings, resentfulness

For each of the roles listed below, pretend the role has been disrupted because of a health problem. Write a possible psychosocial nursing diagnosis, and write a sentence about a situation in which the particular diagnosis you chose would be appropriate. As a critical-thinking exercise, use a different diagnosis for each role alteration. There are a number of different diagnoses that could be appropriate depending on the situation. Note: Students should use the definitions of diagnoses to develop a situation that would reflect the selected diagnosis.

Worker

Nursing Diagnosis: Ineffective Role Performance

Rationale: The health-compromised worker may be unable to perform according to expectations in the work environment.

Student

Nursing Diagnosis: Ineffective Coping

Rationale: The health-compromised student may be unable to appraise stressors in a situation, not be aware of appropriate responses to the situation, or be unable to use available resources in a situation.

Parent

Nursing Diagnosis: Impaired Parenting

Rationale: The parent of a child with a health problem may not be able to create an environment that promotes optimal growth and development of the child.

Husband/wife

Nursing Diagnosis: Sexual Dysfunction

Rationale: Some health problems can lead to unsatisfactory changes in sexual functioning, for example impotence.

Lover

Nursing Diagnosis: Ineffective Sexuality Patterns

Rationale: Some health problems, such as following mastectomy, lead to expressions of concern about difficulties in limitations of sexual behaviors.

Friend

Nursing Diagnosis: Impaired Social Interaction

Rationale: The patient may not be able to participate in sufficient social exchanges or may not feel comfortable in social interactions and may lose a sense of interest in maintaining friendships.

Son/daughter

Nursing Diagnosis: Disabled Family Coping

Rationale: Children of the patient may behave in a manner that disables the ability to effectively address tasks that are essential to the patient's adaptation to the health problem.

Sister/brother

Nursing Diagnosis: Compromised Family Coping

Rationale: A usually supportive sister or brother (family member) is providing insufficient support that may be needed by the patient to manage the health problem.

Grandparent

Nursing Diagnosis: Caregiver Role Strain

Rationale: The grandparent with a role in the care of a grandchild with a health problem may have difficulty in performing roles associated with care of the grandchild.

For each of the psychosocial problems below involving an interaction with the health-care provider, give a psychosocial nursing diagnosis. Write a sentence about why the particular diagnosis you chose would be appropriate. Because this is a critical thinking exercise, use a different diagnosis for each situation.

The patient signs himself out of the hospital against medical advice.

Nursing Diagnosis: Noncompliance

Rationale: The patient is refusing to comply with the therapeutic plan and signs out of the hospital.

The family cannot decide whether or not to permit the patient to have a feeding tube.

Nursing Diagnosis: Decisional Conflict

Rationale: There is a state of uncertainty about the course of action.

The family cannot handle all the care required for the ventilator-dependent child at home.

Nursing Diagnosis: Caregiver Role Strain

Rationale: Caregivers are having difficulty performing their roles in giving care to the child.

The cardiac patient states she has no time to do her exercise prescription.

Nursing Diagnosis: Ineffective Management of Therapeutic Regimen: Individual

Rationale: The patient is having difficulty integrating an exercise prescription into her daily living routines, which compromises specific health goals.

For each of the situations below involving changes in body image or self-esteem, have students give a possible psychosocial nursing diagnosis and write a sentence about why the particular diagnosis chosen would be appropriate. Use a different diagnosis for each alteration. (Note: Only three of the diagnoses deal with body image and self-esteem, so one diagnosis will be duplicated.)

The patient refuses to look at the appendectomy scar.

Nursing Diagnosis: Disturbed Body Image

Rationale: The patient is avoiding looking at the scar. This is an indication of a confused mental picture of one's physical self.

The patient with a heart attack states, "I'm just no good anymore. I'll never be able to go back to my old job."

Nursing Diagnosis: Situational Low Self-Esteem

Rationale: The patient has negative self-evaluation/feelings that developed in response to the heart attack. Before the heart attack, the patient had a positive self-evaluation.

The patient states, "I'm so ashamed of the way I look without my hair since the chemotherapy."

Nursing Diagnosis: Disturbed Body Image

Rationale: The patient is verbalizing feelings of shame about a change in appearance.

The patient states, "I haven't been outside this apartment for six months because I'm a cripple and I don't want anyone to see me."

Nursing Diagnosis: Chronically Low Self-Esteem

Rationale: This patient has longstanding negative self-evaluation and feelings about himself, and is expressing shame in his appearance.

For each of the examples of cultural nursing care problems below, have students give a possible nursing diagnosis and write a sentence about why the particular diagnosis they chose would be appropriate. They should use a different diagnosis for each alteration.

The patient says she can't understand how God could have let this happen to her.

Nursing Diagnosis: Spiritual Distress

Rationale: The patient is questioning her relationship with her God. A principle pervading the person's existence has been disrupted that involves the belief that God must be trusted in all situations and knows what's best.

An East Indian woman comes by ambulance into labor and delivery and screams with each contraction. She doesn't understand English, and there is no interpreter available. Her husband is on the way to the hospital.

Nursing Diagnosis: Impaired Verbal Communication

Rationale: The patient has a language barrier to receive, process, or transmit verbal messages. Communication would be nonverbal only.

The Jehovah's witness with a hemoglobin of 5 is actively bleeding and is refusing blood.

Nursing Diagnosis: Noncompliance

Rationale: The patient is refusing to comply with a treatment that will save his life because of spiritual beliefs. This presents an ethical dilemma for health care providers.

Activity 5

The purpose of this activity is for students to recognize patterns of gender communication in typical situations in health-care settings. Below are gender communication examples. Specify whether they are typical male or female patterns of communication. Tell students to write why they think so and specify what they would say.

The physician comes into the room, says hello, and asks, "What's going on with Mrs. G?" This is a typical male pattern of behavior, and the doctor is asking for a report. The student should report the key assessment data identified in the central box of the concept map care plan.

The nurse says to the patient, "It's time to get up to sit in a chair, don't you think so?" This is a typical female pattern of behavior using a tag question to facilitate harmony, but it makes the nurse asking the question appear uncertain. This tag question could lead to conflict if the patient does not want to get up.

The patient says to the nurse, "I'm sorry to be such a bother to you." This is a typical female pattern of behavior accepting blame for and apologizing for a situation that cannot be avoided and is not the patient's fault. The response is to use empathy to get the patient to verbalize feelings. Make a statement such as, "It is very difficult to be dependent on someone else for help," and wait for a response.

Chapter 7

Concept Maps as the Basis of Documentation

Accurate and precise documentation is very difficult for students to learn. Concept maps are excellent guides for documentation on patient legal records because students easily recognize that everything on the concept map must be documented someplace in the legal records. Students use the concept map diagrams, goals, outcomes, interventions, and patient responses to remind them of all that must be documented. This chapter is focused on relationships among the American Nurses' Association Documentation Standards, Practice Standards, and concept map care plans. Students can use the concept map care plans to guide them in documentation on standardized forms and narrative progress notes. Students must recognize what to document; where to document; and how to write notations legally, accurately, and efficiently.

Teaching Tips

It is very important to emphasize that documentation is part of a legal record, and students are liable for what they do and how they document what was done. Documentation is the legal proof of what happened in the event that the records are subpoenaed in court during malpractice claims. For nurses documentation is the legal proof that nursing standards of care were being followed. Class discussion should focus on *what to document* to provide evidence the nurse:

1. Collected assessment data
2. Analyzed assessment data to determine diagnoses
3. Identified expected patient behavioral outcome objectives
4. Developed a plan with interventions to attain patient behavioral outcome objectives
5. Implemented interventions to attain patient behavioral outcomes
6. Evaluated the patient's progress toward behavioral outcomes.

In addition, teach students that legal records are used for Quality Assurance Audits and evidence of safe and effective delivery of health care. One important criteria health-care agencies must meet to maintain certifications by the Joint Commission of the Accreditation of Health Care Organizations (JCAHO) involves accurate and complete documentation.

Also, students must recognize that billing for services to private insurance agencies, managed care organizations, and government Medicare and Medicaid Services is based on correct documentation. If the documentation is not correct, the health-care agency will not receive appropriate reimbursement for services rendered.

As you teach documentation class, show students *where to document* on flow sheets and clinical narrative progress notes using the concept map care plans as guides. Students can find documentation data to be used in writing on flow sheets and clinical progress notes as follows:

1. Steps 1, 2, and 3 lead to documentation of assessment data supporting diagnoses. Refer to the diagram developed in Steps 1, 2, and 3 when writing abnormal assessment findings. Problems and evidence to support the problems are on the diagram.

2. Step 4 leads to documentation of implementations to attain outcomes. Students write interventions that were done to handle problems.

3. Step 5 leads to documentation of patient responses and progress toward outcome objectives. Students evaluate patients' physical and emotional responses to nursing interventions.

In addition, teach students *how to document* in a legal, concise, and efficient manner by explaining basic documentation rules:

- Make sure the correct patient's name is on each form in the patient's record.
- Use objective and measurable terms about patient behaviors. When summarizing what the patient states, use quotation marks and let the reader draw conclusions.
- Write legibly in black ink.
- Sign first initial, last name, name of school, and student nurse status: D. Lorenzo, YSU, SN.
- Never sign someone else's entry.
- Correct mistakes with one line through incorrect works; never scribble over errors.
- Logically organize information.
- Do not document in advance.
- Write a late entry addendum to progress notes when you've forgotten to document something.
- If you didn't chart it, it wasn't done.
- Write completely and concisely. You can omit *a, the,* and subjects of sentences.
- If a treatment or drug is omitted, it must be explained and documented in the progress notes.
- Progress notes must include any discussions of patient care with other health-care providers.
- Never write critical comments about other health-care providers.

Learning Activities: Rationales and Sample Answers

Activity 1

The purpose of correcting charting examples is to give students practice in documentation. The following are charting examples taken from actual medical records. For each entry, what needs to be done to correct it? Correct answers are indicated in boldface.

By the time he was admitted, his rapid heart had stopped, and he was feeling better. **The patient reports he had a "rapid heart rate" prior to admission.**

Patient has chest pain if she lies on her left side for over a year. **The patient reports chest pain when lying on her left side, which has occurred for more than 1 year.**

She has had no rigors or shaking chills, but her husband says she was very hot in bed last night. **Patient's husband reports the patient had a temperature during the night, denies witnessing shaking chills.**

The patient has been depressed since she began seeing me in 1993. **The patient has a history of depression since 1993.**

I have suggested that he loosen his pants before standing, so that when he stands with the help of his wife, they fall to the floor. **Patient and spouse given instructions for dressing self-care deficit.**

Healthy appearing decrepit 69-year-old male, mentally alert but forgetful. **69-year-old male, alert and oriented to person, place, and time. Reports being "forgetful."** (Healthy appearance needs to be described in terms of age, gender, LOC, skin color and facial expression. There is not enough assessment data to proceed further with this documentation.)

Patient has left his white blood cells at another hospital. **The patient reports he forgot to obtain the WBC report before he left ______(name) hospital.**

The patient refused an autopsy. **The patient's family refused an autopsy.**

The patient is tearful and crying constantly. She also appears to be depressed. **The patient is tearful and crying. She states " …."**

Large brown stool ambulating in the hall. **Patient was incontinent of a large brown stool while ambulating in the hall.**

Skin: somewhat pale but present. **Skin pale.**

Patient has two teenage children but no other abnormalities. **Two teenage children.**

The patient had waffles for breakfast and anorexia for lunch. **The patient ate __% of breakfast, ___% of lunch.**

She slipped on ice, and her legs went in separate directions in early December. **Patient reports she fell on the ice in early December (date). She reports injury to her legs (describe damage).**

Discharge status: Alive but without permission. **Patient left hospital without permission of his/her physician.**

Patient released to the outpatient department without dressing. **Patient accompanied to the outpatient department by _______. Refused to dress in street clothing because_______.**

The patient expired on the floor uneventfully. **Breathing and heartbeat ceased at _____.**

The patient has no past history of suicides. **The patient denies attempting suicide**.

Since she can't get pregnant without her husband, I thought you would like to work her up. **Referred to _______ for infertility studies.**

The patient will need disposition, and therefore we will get Dr. Smith to dispose of him. **Will contact Dr. Smith for discharge orders.**

Activity 2

Practice writing narrative PIE statements for the concept map care plan of the patient with diabetes from Chapter 5 using Figure 5–1. There are two problems that would require PIE documentation; the other items would be documented on flow sheets.

Sample 1

0735 Imbalanced Nutrition: Blood sugar 60, diaphoretic, appears anxious. Reports feeling dizzy and hungry. P. O'Brien, YSU, SN --

0735 Patient given breakfast and drank orange juice. Notified Mrs. Campo, RN. P. O'Brien, YSU, SN---

0750 Ate 90% breakfast. Patient states "feels much better." Skin warm and dry. P. O'Brien, YSU, SN---

O800 Insulin held, Dr. notified, will call Dr. for further orders after next Accu-check.

Sample 2

1015 Deficient knowledge: Signs and symptoms of hyperglycemia and hypoglycemia, insulin administration, use of Accu-check discussed and demonstrated. Needs continued practice with Accu-check. Did not need 0800 insulin so could not practice self-administration. Was able to correctly draw up medication. Can state the signs of hypoglycemia and hyperglycemia. Review of diabetic menus not done because of lack of time. P. O'Brien, YSU, SN--------------

1100 Diabetic educator visited and patient scheduled to start classes when discharged at the outpatient clinic. P. O'Brien, YSU, SN---

Chapter 8

After the Clinical Day Is Done: Patient Evaluations and Self-evaluations

After the clinical day is done, the student needs to complete evaluation of patient outcomes and performance self-evaluations. Students can complete patient evaluations and self-evaluations of clinical performance in approximately 30 to 60 minutes. Grading concept map care plans is not difficult because they have been used by the students and critiqued by you throughout the clinical day. You have already reviewed the concept map care plans except for the students' evaluations of patients' progress toward goals and objectives. Grading concept map care plans can be done quickly because of your familiarity with the concept map care plans and because the information is concisely organized.

This chapter's primary focus in the identification of the relationship between standards of nursing performance related to patient evaluations and self-evaluations . Students need to understand the role of faculty in providing performance evaluations to help students grow into their professional roles. In foundations courses, students need to be introduced to the purposes of performance evaluations and to learn how to appropriately behave in response to a performance evaluation by clinical faculty. Many students have never had a performance evaluation done prior to enrollment in a nursing program.

Teaching Tips

The students need to understand the purpose of performance evaluations. In foundations classes, I have noted that at least half the students have never had one before. Teach that purposes of performance evaluations are to accomplish three basic objectives:

1. To determine if safe and effective care is provided.

2. To determine grades.

3. To determine if students should be promoted to the next course.

Students need to understand that performance evaluations are both formative and summative. *Formative evaluations* are done on a weekly basis to evaluate progress towards specific daily clinical objectives. *Summative evaluations* are done at midterm and the completion of the term to summarize performance abilities related to course objectives. Review sample clinical site objectives and course objectives as you explain the purpose of performance evaluations. Explain specific clinical expectations using the clinical objectives so that students are aware of responsibilities regarding patient care and that patient safety is always the priority.

Emphasize that if they are not sure of what to do or have not learned it yet, they should inform you and the staff nurse who is responsible for patient care. Also review your school's dismissal policy for unsafe behaviors.

A very important aspect of safe and effective professional nursing practice is the need for an objective self-evaluation. Therefore, sample weekly performance evaluation tools provided in this chapter include space for both student and faculty evaluative comments. Have the students turn in the self-evaluations with their concept map care plans on a weekly basis. By reviewing the self-evaluations, you can easily determine whether you and students hold similar or differing views about weekly performance. In using this tool, there are many times when I have been surprised that students thought nothing of what I thought was a major violation of safety, or students have been very hard on themselves and have engaged in self-recriminations.

As students learn about self-evaluations, they must learn what to do if they make a mistake. They need reassurance that everyone makes mistakes and that no one is perfect. It is part of human nature to make them. There are three important things to focus teaching on when (not if) professional nurses or professional student nurses make mistakes:

1. Accept responsibility and own the mistake. Don't make excuses. Admit you were wrong.

2. Never purposely cover up an error. If you attempt to cover an error, you are indicating that you can't be trusted.

3. Don't beat yourself up with self-recriminations such as, "I am very stupid." Instead focus on the behavior you need to improve. For example: "I am intelligent. I wouldn't have made it this far if I wasn't. I made a mistake and won't do it again."

Because many students have never had a performance evaluation prior to entering nursing school, students must be given an explanation of how to take a performance evaluation. Start by explaining that faculty will constructively criticize student performance. The purpose of the criticism is to give the student objective feedback about clinical behaviors and to help students grow into professional roles. Emphasize the following points when teaching students how to take a performance evaluation:

- View criticism from faculty as being given with helpful intent.
- Listen to your faculty's perspective, and avoid offering excuses.
- Ask for clarification and examples of inappropriate behavior.
- Check for mutual understanding, summarizing behaviors that must be changed.
- Ask for help and support in areas of future growth.

In addition to giving performance evaluations, faculty need to assign grades to patient profile databases, concept map care plans, and teaching plans. I recommend separate letter grades for each component of the written requirements so that students can determine components of concept map care plans they are doing well and components they need to improve.

Assign a letter grade to:

1. Combine patient profile database, pressure sore assessment, and falls risk assessments
2. Concept map diagram—Steps 1, 2, and 3.
3. Goals, objectives, and interventions—Step 4
4. Evaluation of patient responses and clinical impressions—Step 5
5. Documentation on legal records
6. Method teaching plan and evaluation of teaching

Although there are six grades to be completed, you will find that grading takes less time because information is better organized and you have already reviewed and critiqued concept map care plans throughout the clinical day.

Rationales for Learning Activities

Activity 1

Analysis of objectives from two sequential clinical nursing courses helps students to focus on comparing similarities and differences in nursing knowledge to be learned with related performance expectations. Students should identify evidence of American Nurses Association standards of clinical nursing practice in course objectives. They should also recognize that nursing knowledge is sequentially expanded from course to course. Course objectives are the basis for self-evaluations and faculty evaluations of student cognitive knowledge and clinical performance.

Activity 2

The purpose of analysis of clinical site behavioral objectives is for students to recognize the relationship between the course objectives and the site objectives. The clinical site objectives involve the day-to-day objectives that are carefully planned for each clinical experience. Student strengths and weaknesses are summarized in a formative manner by faculty and students as they go from week to week, and in a summative manner at midterm and at completion of the course. Give examples of strengths and weaknesses to help students understand the nature of clinical evaluations.

Activity 3

Reviewing your school's dismissal policy for unsafe clinical practice emphasizes student weaknesses that may result in dismissal from the nursing program. By comparing your school's policy with the sample policy in this book, students recognize similarities in dismissal policies based on universal principles of protecting the safety of patients.

Author's Note

I wish you well in teaching nursing students how to plan, implement, and evaluate care. It is an awesome responsibility. I have enjoyed presenting clinical concept map care plans at conferences and workshops around the country, and I hope to continue to do so. Faculty have responded enthusiastically, and I have heard from a number of faculty as they integrate concept map care plans into courses. I consider concept map care plans to be continually evolving as they are adapted into different levels of nursing curriculums. I would like to have your critique of this new method of care planning. Please send comments, questions, and concerns about care planning to me via e-mail at paschust@cc.ysu.edu, or you may write to me at Youngstown State University, Department of Nursing, Youngstown, Ohio 44555.

